P9-EDK-154

Investigating Recreational and Commercial Diving Accidents

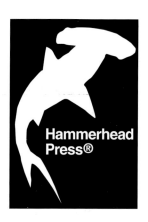

Hammerhead
Press®

by
Steven M. Barsky
and
Tom Neuman, M.D., FACP, FACPM

© Copyright 2003 Steven M. Barsky and Tom Neuman. All rights reserved.

No part of this book may be reproduced or transmitted in any form or by any means electronic or mechanical, including photocopying, recording, or by any information storage or retrieval system, without permission in writing from the publisher.

Original photography and illustrations by Steven M. Barsky unless otherwise noted. Design and typography by Hammerhead Press

Cover photo © 2003 Bob Evans / La Mer Bleu Productions

Printing history: First printing 2003

Printed in the United States of America by Ojai Printing, Ojai, California.

ISBN Number: 0-9674305-3-4

Library of Congress Card Catalog Number: 2003110690

Other Books by Steven M. Barsky

Published by Best Publishing
Careers in Diving
The Simple Guide to Rebreather Diving
The Simple Guide to Snorkeling Fun
Small Boat Diving
Spearfishing for Skin and Scuba Divers

Published by Hammerhead Press
Diving in High-Risk Environments, Third Edition
Dry Suit Diving, Third Edition
California Lobster Diving (with Kristine Barsky)

Published by International Training, Inc.
Deeper Sport Diving with Dive Computers
Easy Nitrox Diving
Underwater Navigation, Night, and Limited Visibility Diving
Wreck, Boat, and Drift Diving

Published by Scuba Schools International
The Dry Suit Diving Manual

Other Books by
Tom Neuman, M.D., FACP, FACPM
The Physiology and Medicine of Diving (Neuman and Brubakk, Editors)

Table of Contents

Table of Contents

Table of Contents

Table of Contents

Acknowledgements

As always, I have relied on numerous people to assist me in reviewing the manuscript for technical accuracy and assisting me in innumerable ways. I am indebted to the following people for their assistance:

• Former commercial diver, and current diving safety officer, Gary Beyerstein graciously allowed us to use his photographs of the helicopter crash that took place on the derrick barge Thor in the North Sea in the 1970s. Gary and I worked together on several diving jobs and he always took the time to help me when I was a tender in the industry.

• Underwater photographer and diver Pete Nawrocky allowed us to use one of his photos of a technical diver in action.

• Lt. Dave Jephson of the Terrace Water Rescue Team in Canada shared several of his photos of search and rescue divers in action.

• Photographer and friend, Bob Evans, shot the cover photo for us and provided other photography. Bob is a true creative genius.

• Donna Wyatt at Texas Research Institute (TRI) provided assistance with air sampling apparatus. TRI is one of the leaders in air sampling services for the diving industry.

• Former Los Angeles County Sheriff's Commander and friend Mike Quinn reviewed the manuscript for accuracy. I will always be personally indebted to Mike for taking the time to teach me how to teach scuba diving when I was just a teenager, and for his friendship.

• Former commercial diver and friend Bob Christensen has always come to our aid whenever we have asked for help. Bob read the manuscript and made numerous suggestions for improvement. Bob has been one of the most important mentors in my life.

• Attorney and diver Laura Horton, with whom I have worked on many cases, reviewed the legal accuracy of this book. Laura has guided me through many legal cases and has always been available for help when I need it. Her extensive experience and wisdom in dealing with many diving cases has always been invaluable.

• Nick Fanelli, friend and Vice-President at General Star Management, read the book and shared his insights on the insurance industry's perspective on diving accidents. Nick was the first person to give me the chance to investigate diving accidents on a professional basis.

• Lt. Jim Elliott of the U.S. Coast Guard provided a comprehensive technical review of the work with his unique perspective from the field. Jim is the recipient of the U.S. Coast Guard's commendation medal for spearheading the in-depth field investigations of commercial diving accidents in the Gulf of Mexico.

Finally, both Tom and I thank our wives, Doris and Kristine respectively, for providing us with the time and support to complete this project.

Steve Barsky
Ventura, California

Introduction

I have always considered myself an advocate for sport diving as well as commercial diving, particularly for the individual diver and the industries that support both the sport and professions of diving. Without the diving equipment manufacturers and service providers who work in these industries, there would be no diving as we know it today.

When a diving fatality or serious diving accident takes place, there is always intense interest in the local diving community as to what happened and why. Unfortunately, there is also often wild speculation, which sometimes leads to recriminations, as folks assign blame or make assumptions about the facts of the matter. The Internet, which is a wonderful forum for the communication of facts and information, has also been a breeding ground for individuals to post their personal theories on incidents about which they have no personal knowledge. In our society, the parties involved are usually advised to remain silent about what happened, which may lead to further speculation.

Like most divers, I too have always been interested in the causes of diving accidents and this interest has in large part shaped my career. In college, I studied human factors/ergonomics including applied anatomy and took a special interest in the design of diving equipment, diving physiology, and diver performance. However, it was not until many years later that I had the opportunity to combine the various aspects of my career into the formal investigation of diving accidents.

After working as a diving instructor, dive guide, and commercial diver, I had the good fortune to work for Diving Systems International (now Kirby Morgan Diving Systems) in Santa Barbara from 1983-1986. I then worked for Viking, the dry suit equipment manufacturer, for two years before starting my own company, Marine Marketing and Consulting. Through publication, I became involved in expert witness work in diving accident litigation, and began investigating diving accidents for insurance companies in the early 1990s.

My diving accident investigations have taken me throughout the United States, Mexico, and the Dominican Republic. This is not happy work, but I have derived a certain fulfillment from knowing that I have helped to reduce the risks in diving as a result of my investigations. The work you are reading here is the end product of handling diving accident investigations for several major insurance companies and numerous attorneys.

This book is not concerned with specific underwater forensic techniques. Officer Robert Teather of the Royal Canadian Mounted Police has already written an excellent book on that topic, that focuses on the underwater crime scene, body recovery, and similar topics. Rather, this book spotlights the human interactions that take place prior to, during, and after a diving accident, the detailed examination of diving equipment, analysis of the dive site, analysis of medical reports, and a review of training factors.

It has become apparent to me that in most cases, the recovery of the victim of a fatal diving accident is usually handled by the divers who are at the site at the time of the accident. Consequently, a good investigation requires an investigator who is skilled at interviewing people, has a detailed knowledge of diving equipment and procedures, and the capability to take this information and put it together into a coherent report.

Most individuals who work in the diving profession are extremely safety conscious and have done a good job of reducing the number of accidents in their businesses. While we probably can never reduce the number of diving accidents to zero, we can always look for new ways to improve safety.

The addition of Tom Neuman, M.D., FACP, FACPM as a co-author of this book provides a wealth of insight to diving accidents from a medical and practical perspective. As a former Navy doctor and diver, a diving medical officer, a sport diver, and the operator of the U.C. San Diego Hyperbaric Medical Center, Tom brings a unique and learned perspective to this work. His participation in the San Diego coroner's committee that investigates diving deaths has put him in direct contact with law enforcement personnel, lifeguards, and diving instructors who must put the pieces together when a diving accident takes place.

Together, we hope that our combined experience will assist you in helping to make diving safer for everyone and in conducting your dive accident investigations.

Steven Barsky
Ventura, California

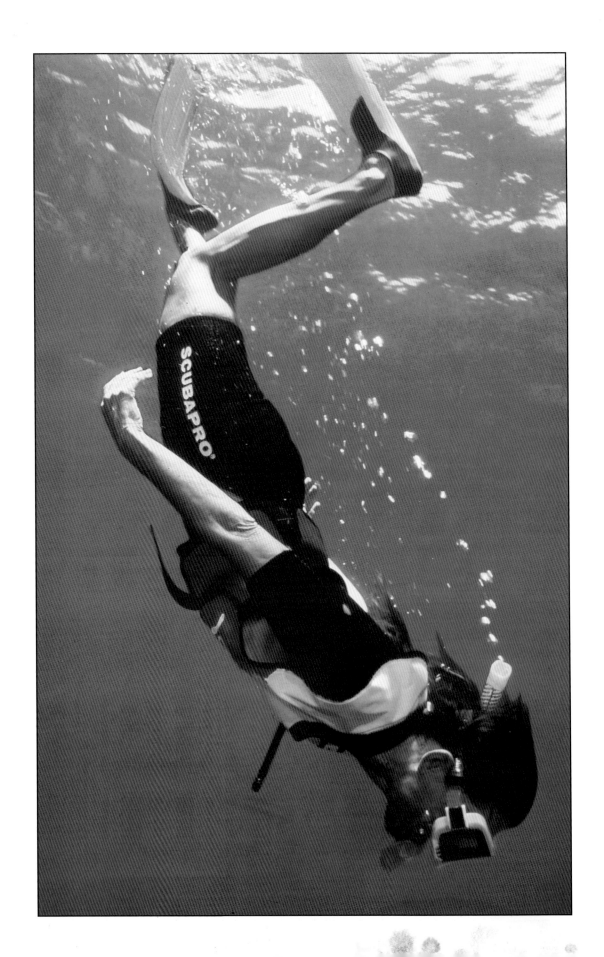

Chapter 1
Why Investigate Diving Accidents?

When people go underwater, whether it is for recreation or work, there is always the potential they may be injured or killed. Even the most beautiful coral reef located near a "tropical paradise" must be considered a potentially hostile environment, because whenever people dive, accidents are always possible.

In recreational diving, people go underwater to have fun. The training that they receive in their initial diver training course normally includes the basic skills for survival underwater. In most cases, this training is not enough to produce a proficient diver. Only through repeated practice and numerous dives under a variety of conditions does a diver begin to accumulate the knowledge, judgement, and comfort level in the water to handle challenging conditions underwater.

For the purposes of this book, "technical diving" has been included under the heading of recreational diving. In technical diving, people use advanced equipment to reach extreme depths or extend their bottom time beyond what is considered normal for recreational diving. However, the purpose of technical diving is still recreation, i.e., the diver is not being paid for his time underwater.

Between the recreational diver and the hard-core commercial diver lies another category of diver that could be called the "professional diver." These are people who work underwater, but are not involved in operations such as heavy construction or salvage, and do not have the level of support found in most commercial diving operations. This group might

include public safety divers, professional underwater photographers, marine biologists and archaeologists, seafood divers, and others involved in similar occupations. They are paid to go underwater and perform work, but their tools are usually cameras, collecting nets, rakes, or similar items. Their training usually exceeds that of the sport diver, but does not match that of the commercial diver.

In commercial diving, people go underwater to perform heavy work, usually involving some type of tool, and frequently under demanding conditions. Like recreational diving, the commercial

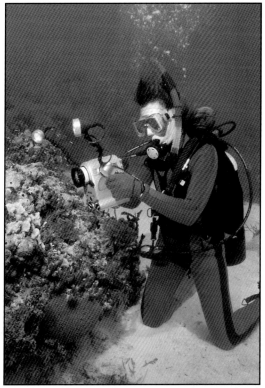

Fig. 1.1 All diving has a certain degree of risk involved.

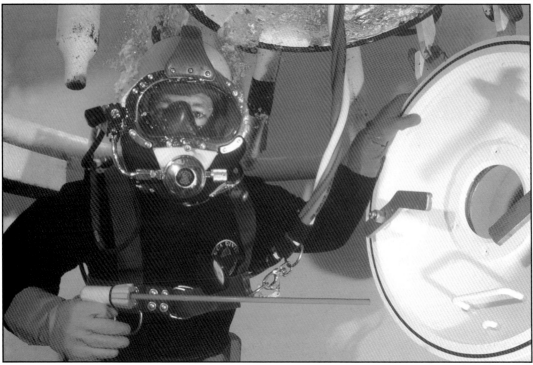

Fig. 1.2 Commercial divers go underwater to do many different types of work.

diver's training is usually only sufficient to produce a novice diver. In the commercial world, the novice diver is known as a "tender,"; i.e., a person with sufficient training to allow them to function as an apprentice. It usually takes several years before a new commercial diver has adequate experience and judgement to know what they can and cannot do and when it is wiser to decline to make a dive.

Recreational and commercial diving accidents occur for a variety of reasons. People are human and make mistakes, placing themselves in situations that exceed their training, their personal limitations, and the limitations of their equipment. Divers experience "undeserved" cases of decompression sickness, unprovoked lung over-expansion injuries, and heart attacks that just happen to occur while they are diving. Equipment can fail unexpectedly and weather and sea conditions can change dramatically. External factors, such as boats that suddenly cross through the dive site, can also contribute to injuries and fatalities.

In many cases, there is no one single factor that triggers a diving accident, but a variety of individual contributing elements that collectively add up to a mishap which usually could have been prevented. When this unfortunate combination of events occurs, the final trigger may obscure the underlying events that had to take place before the accident would happen.

Accident Investigations Satisfy Needs

Diving accident investigations satisfy the diverse needs of different people and various organizations in different ways. While these investigations may focus on specific aspects of an accident, the reports generated by dive accident investigators will usually have many similarities.

At the most basic level, an accident investigation will help to identify why a particular injury or fatality took place. This information will frequently be used to help create regulations or procedures that will help prevent this type of accident in the future. Investigations will often identify a weak point in training, procedures, or equipment.

Law enforcement authorities with very different responsibilities typically approach diving accidents as though a crime has been committed. Until a death has been investigated, it is usually impossible to know why it has occurred. In many jurisdictions, diving accidents are treated as homicides until proven otherwise.

Another indirect result of dive accident investigations is to satisfy the family's need to know about the cause of death of a loved one. While this is rarely the prime motivation for an investigation, it is one of the more satisfying end results of an inquiry of this type.

Other Types of Investigations

Insurance companies that write policies for dive stores and diving instructors routinely investigate diving accidents. The purpose of these investigations is to collect the facts and document the evidence in the case. These investigations are done under the assumption that litigation will be filed against the insured store or instructor. Attorney-client privilege may extend to the investigator in these cases.

The United States Coast Guard may investigate diving accidents to ensure that there have been no violations of the commercial diving regulations, rules of the road, or safe boating practices. OSHA, the Occupational Safety and Health Administration, also conducts investigations into some commercial diving accidents. They have their own set of regulations and may levy fines on violators of the OSHA standards.

Litigation frequently occurs following a diving accident, where the family of the deceased or the injured diver attempts to recover damages from the party they believe to be responsible for the injury. Attorneys for plaintiffs may hire their own investigators and/or experts to try to determine the cause of the accident to decide whether they are able to prove "damage" or wrongful death.

Putting Dive Accidents in Perspective

In an average year, there are usually 90-110 sport diving fatalities in the United States, plus many more non-fatal diving accidents such as decompression sickness. The Divers Alert Network (DAN) maintains records on diving accidents and distributes an annual report on fatalities each year.

It's difficult to put this figure in per-

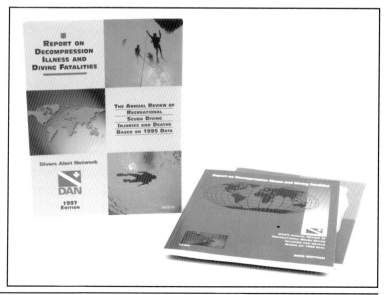

Fig. 1.3 The Divers Alert Network issues an annual report on diving fatalities.

Risk Recognition for Divers and Diving Professionals

If you are professionally employed in diving, be it recreational or commercial, you may, at some point in your life, be involved in a diving accident. The longer you teach diving, or the more commercial diving jobs you perform, the greater the odds are that you will witness or be caught up in the emotional trauma surrounding an injury or fatality. The minute details of the circumstances surrounding the accident will be scrutinized at the microscopic level.

To have a complete record of your actions it is essential to be sure that you complete and maintain all of the paperwork that surrounds your business. This includes, but is not limited to, the following:

- Waivers and releases
- Training records
- Applications for employment and/or training
- Records of personnel testing and/or training
- Equipment maintenance records and receipts
- Air samples
- Sales receipts
- Dive logs
- Physical exam forms

In the event of an accident, you will be asked to produce these documents and in all probability, many others. When an investigation takes place, these records will help to verify what took place in your operation prior to the incident .

---

spective because the exact number of divers there are in the U.S., or the number of dives they make each year are unknown. There is no central registry of divers, nor any government mandated logbook requirement as there is for aircraft pilots.

Current statistics from the U.S. Sporting Goods Manufacturers Association puts the number of active recreational divers in the U.S. at approximately 2.25-2.5 million divers. If the "average" diver makes approximately 12 dives per year, then it would appear that the number of fatal accidents is approximately one per 200,000 dives.

Scientific divers track the number of accidents among their ranks rather carefully and they have an extremely good safety record. Their organization, the AAUS (American Academy of Underwater Sciences) maintains high training standards and has requirements for routine diving physicals and recertification of their members. It is highly unusual for a scientific diver to die as a result of a div-

ing accident.

Unfortunately, it is much more difficult to know the total number of accidents for most other types of diving. There is no published annual report on deaths or serious injuries among professional divers, such as seafood divers or public safety divers, although sometimes these incidents are included in DAN's reports. Although OSHA collects statistics on these incidents when the information comes to their attention, they do not have the resources to proactively collect this type of data. Similarly, the statistics on commercial diving accidents are difficult to come by.

Financial Costs of Diving Accidents

The financial costs of even a sport diving accident, whether fatal or non-fatal, can be astronomical. Many different agencies may respond to a diving accident, with varying levels of involvement.

When a diving accident occurs at a

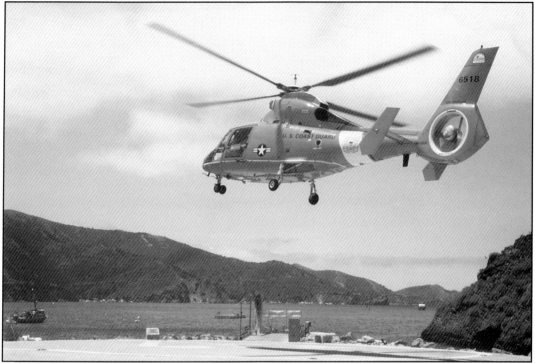

Fig. 1.4 The U.S. Coast Guard is usually the first agency to respond when an accident takes place at a remote location off the coast of the United States.

remote location off the coast of the U.S., the first agency that will usually respond is the U.S. Coast Guard. They will usually mobilize a rescue helicopter with a crew of four. Although they do not bill the public for their response to life threatening emergencies, you can imagine what it must cost to operate these aircraft.

If the accident takes place close to shore, or on the beach, the diver may still require an air ambulance if he needs treatment in a hyperbaric chamber and there is no facility close-by. Air ambulance costs run thousands of dollars per hour and not all insurance policies cover diving accidents.

If the diver is taken to a hyperbaric chamber for treatment, these facilities also operate at a high cost. Most chambers today are associated with hospitals and patients, or their families, are billed for all items used in treatment as well as for medical personnel who attend them. Some insurance policies do not cover diving accidents. Although some people

make dramatic recoveries from diving accidents, other people may need extended treatment or physical therapy.

Aside from the direct costs of dealing with a diving accident, there are also the costs of lost wages as a result of the death of a family provider, the cost of investigating the accident, and the cost of litigation, if it occurs.

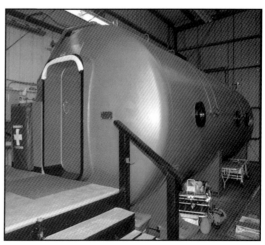

Fig. 1.5 Treatment in a hyperbaric chamber is time consuming and expensive.

Human Costs of Diving Accidents

While the financial costs of a dive accident are almost always high, the human costs are frequently higher. The loss of a loved one is irreparable.

For a sport diving instructor who has lost a student, or a commercial diving supervisor who has lost a diver, the toll in lost sleep and self-doubt can be overwhelming. It takes some people many years, if ever, before they can approach these situations with any degree of normalcy again. If litigation follows the accident, the human toll on all those involved escalates. In addition, should an individual be chronically incapacitated, or a child injured or killed, marriages may dissolve with all the attendant hardship associated with divorce.

The investigation, depositions, and courtroom testimony force the survivors to relive the incident over and over again. Even if the persons involved did nothing wrong, every action and response they made will be scrutinized and questioned. It is a distinctly unpleasant experience for everyone who was present during the event.

Your Dive Accident Investigation

No matter what your purpose in investigating diving accidents, the basic approach will be the same. Certain techniques, procedures, and elements are common to all dive accident investigations.

Almost all dive accident investigations take place days or even weeks after the incident. In many instances, by the time the investigator gets involved, the body will already have been recovered, the equipment disassembled, and the witnesses dispersed to their homes. Unless the case is a fatality and the investigator was part of the team who helped to recover the body, the investigator will nearly always be dependent on the observations of others.

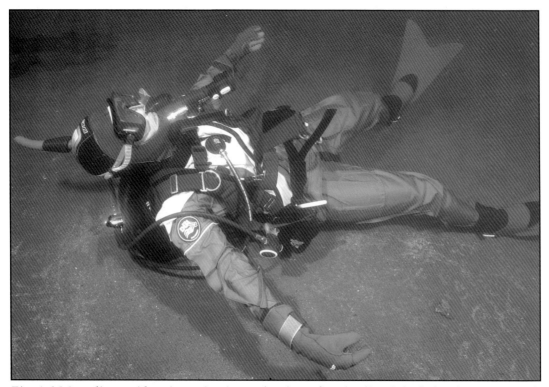

Fig. 1.6 Most dive accident investigations take place after the diver's body has been recovered.

Case History – Recreational Diving Accident

A female diver who was previously certified through a dive store, signed up to take an advanced diving class through the same store. She completed the open-water training for the basic course, but during one of the pool sessions, had an incident occur where she passed out briefly in the pool. The instructor was beside her during the incident and she was immediately revived.

The instructor attributed the incident to the weather, which was extremely warm, and allowed the student to continue the course and become certified. The student was never referred to a physician for examination following the incident.

During one of the advanced open water dives, the student became separated from her buddy and was later found dead on the bottom. In the course of the investigation, the incident during the first open water course was revealed. Subsequently, the store owner made mention that the student was thought to have rented some equipment from another local store.

The investigator traveled to the second store, where information was provided by the second store owner that the student had enrolled in a specialty diving course through his facility. A copy of the diver's student folder at the second store was provided. On the medical statement form the student indicated that she had been taking a prescription drug, Effexor, which is usually prescribed for depression. Side effects of the drug may include dizziness, impaired motor skills, and impaired judgment, all of which could obviously be serious underwater. Equally important, the diagnosis of depression is also critical when investigating an otherwise unexplained diving death. The student never revealed this information to the original dive store and the second store owner had missed this information.

If the second store had not been visited, this vital information would probably never have been discovered. This is just one example of the importance of following up on all potential information that you encounter during an investigation.

Note that with the passage of the Health Insurance Portability and Accountability Act (HIPAA) which went into effect in April of 2003, the collection and dissemination of medical information most likely will be more restricted. This will have a profound effect on investigations and provides for criminal penalties for violations of the law. It will also probably impact the medical history information that sport diving instructors may collect on their prospective students.

This book will help you to learn the procedures you need to conduct effective and complete dive accident investigations. There is no great mystery to this type of work, but you do need to have a better than average understanding of diving equipment, physiology, techniques, and procedures. You also must be tenacious in pursuing every piece of information relating to the incidents you investigate. The skills that you will need to be a successful investigator will be explored in detail in other parts of this book.

While some people come by these skills and talents easily, others will have to apply themselves to develop the ability to produce professional quality reports. As with most things in life, it all boils down to a question of effort and desire, and how important it is to you to be successful in this field.

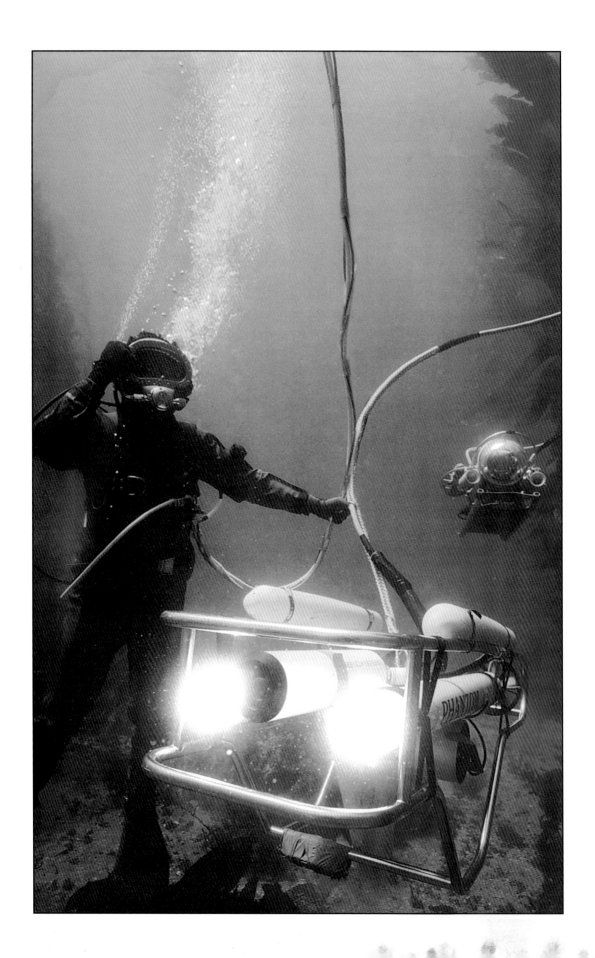

Chapter 2
Modes of Diving

There are several different "modes" of diving as we've already discussed, and this usually refers to the procedures and the type of equipment that the diver is using.

Newspaper accounts of diving accidents are often inaccurate and frequently confuse the type of diving in which the victim was engaged at the time of the accident. It is not uncommon for a newspaper to refer to a scuba diver as a "skin diver."

The equipment used during a dive will normally depend on the purpose, depth, and location of the dive. The type of equipment does not determine the type of diving that is being done. In certain circumstances, a scientific diver, a public safety diver, and a commercial diver all might use exactly the same type of equipment.

In recreational diving there are two modes that are normally used, i.e., breath-hold diving and the use of self contained underwater breathing apparatus (scuba). Professional divers, including scientists and public-safety divers, may use either scuba gear or a helmet with breathing gas supplied from the surface. Commercial divers almost always use a helmet with the breathing gas pumped down through a hose from the surface.

In commercial diving, there are several different variations of the equipment and procedures that might be followed, such as the use of a diving bell or what's

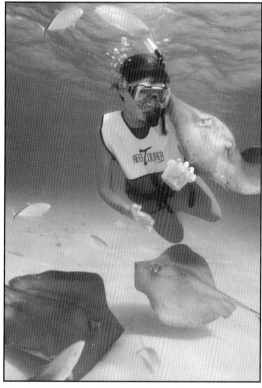

Fig. 2.1 Breath-hold diving is just one type of recreational diving.

known as a "saturation system." However, in almost all instances, the basic system is dependent on breathing gas supplied to the diver from the surface via a hose. Hence the term, "surface-supplied diving."

In this chapter, the different modes of diving will be examined including snorkeling, breath-hold diving, scuba, surface-supplied, bell diving, and saturation diving.

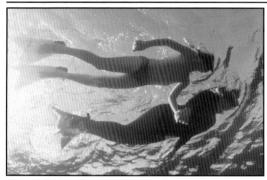

Fig. 2.2 People who engage in snorkeling may never go below the surface of the water. (© Bob Evans/La Mer Bleu. All rights reserved.)

Snorkeling

Snorkeling is the least sophisticated type of "diving." In fact, some snorkelers never actually go underwater, but simply paddle around on the surface and observe things underwater from there. Almost all snorkeling is done for recreational purposes. Many snorkelers use the least expensive gear they can find, often purchased at discount centers, ordinary sporting goods stores (as opposed to specialty dive shops), and resort gift shops. Sometimes, this type of equipment is poorly manufactured.

Skin Diving or Free Diving

Skin diving is also called "breath-hold diving," which is a more descriptive term and leaves less possibility for confusion. In this type of diving, the diver does not wear any type of breathing apparatus other than a snorkel, mask, and fins and possibly a weight belt or personal flotation device. The snorkel is used to allow the diver to float on the surface with his face in the water and breathe without the need to lift his head to take a breath. Any diving made below the surface is accomplished by the person holding his breath.

There are many serious skin divers who take great pride in their ability to hold their breath and dive to great depths or for extended periods underwater. Most serious spearfishing is done by divers holding their breath, since the bubbles released by scuba equipment may frighten many of the more prized game fish.

Most skin diving is done solely for recreation. Serious skin divers tend to use the same basic equipment as scuba divers (mask, fins, and snorkel) and their gear is usually of good quality.

A competent skin diver can dive to depths of 100 feet or more, holding his breath, although the average person usually does not dive deeper than 20 or 30 feet.

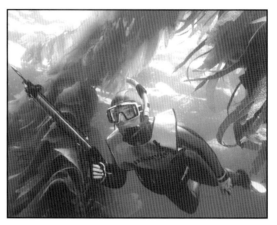

Fig. 2.3 Competent skin divers can reach depths of 100 feet or more.

Scuba Diving

The word "scuba" is actually an "acronym," a word where each letter in the word stands for another word. Scuba stands for "self-contained underwater breathing apparatus." However, the word has become part of the common language of everyday use and the word scuba is now used to refer to anything that has to do with sport diving, as in "scuba travel," "scuba boat," etc.

In most cases, scuba divers use ordinary compressed air for their diving, but there are also divers who use other gas mixtures and specialized equipment. Scuba gear is used by many divers for recreation, but it is also used professionally. Scuba gear is used by scientists, law enforcement and other public safety divers, and for "light" commercial diving.

When most people think of scuba diving, they think of traditional "open-circuit" scuba gear, where the diver breathes compressed air in and exhales through the regulator directly into the water. Actually, when a reference is made to scuba diving, any type of self-contained breathing apparatus, including devices known as "rebreathers" could be meant.

Rebreathers differ from open-circuit scuba in that the rebreather "recycles" the diver's exhaled breath, "scrubs out" (chemically removes) the carbon dioxide, and replenishes the oxygen. Although only a small percentage of the sport diving population uses rebreathers, they have become increasingly popular over the last few years. The two main types of rebreathers that the accident investigator may encounter are semi-closed circuit and fully-closed circuit. The differences between rebreathers will be examined in the chapter on equipment.

Whether a diver uses open-circuit scuba or a rebreather, he is still a "scuba" diver if he carries his entire life support system (i.e. breathing gas supply) with him underwater.

Scuba equipment is rarely used for any serious type of commercial diving operation. It is not generally considered

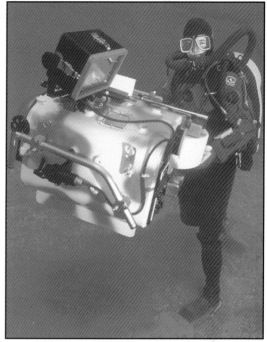

Fig. 2.4 This rebreather is classified as a closed-circuit scuba system.

a viable mode for producing any real useful work, due to its limited air supply and lack of communications.

Scuba Certifications

In the United States, there is no legal requirement for a diver to be certified in the sport of scuba diving. However, the

---

Risk Recognition for Divers and Diving Professionals

Pure oxygen is widely recognized today as the de facto standard for first aid in almost all diving accidents, but especially in cases of arterial gas embolism and decompression sickness. This applies to both recreational and commercial diving accidents.

On the recreational side, although most of the diver training agencies in the world do not have a standard that requires a diving professional to carry an oxygen administration system with them, the prudent diving instructor will do so whenever he is teaching, either in the pool or in an open water situation. Although most dive boats carry oxygen systems on board, given the relatively low cost involved in owning such a system, every instructor should be equipped with this gear.

In the commercial diving world, the need for oxygen in the event of an accident is just as vital. Fortunately, oxygen is almost always on hand whenever a decompression chamber is present on a diving job, but there are some jobs that go out that do not require a chamber and where no oxygen is present. Again, when the low cost of an oxygen system is balanced against its possible benefit, there is no excuse for not having oxygen on every commercial diving operation.

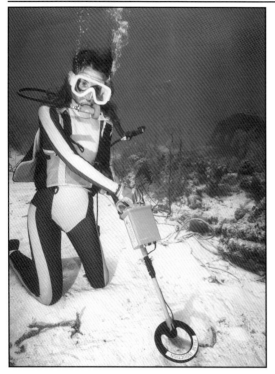

Fig. 2.5 Recreational divers have widely vary-ing levels of expertise. This diver is using a metal detector to locate a shipwreck.

industry voluntarily cooperates in polic-ing itself by requiring proof of diver train-ing in the form of a "certification card" before providing services to divers and before selling certain types of equipment.

Within the sport of scuba diving, div-ers may have various levels of expertise. An entry-level diver is considered an "open water scuba diver." There are also specialty courses, in a wide variety of top-ics, that divers may take after completing their initial certification. These courses cover such diverse topics as night diving, underwater photography, and ice diving.

Leadership levels in diving include certifications such as divemaster, assis-tant instructor, instructor, and instruc-tor-trainer. Of course, the experience and expertise of the people involved in the training of divers can vary greatly.

At the extreme end of the recreational diving field is the "technical diver." Tech-nical diving generally involves dives that are deeper and/or longer than ordinary

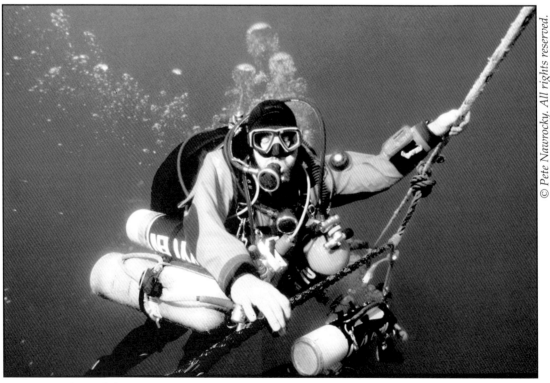

© Pete Nawrocky. All rights reserved.

Fig. 2.6 Technical divers usually wear and carry multiple scuba cylinders so they can switch breathing gases on deep dives. They regularly practice solo diving and strive for complete self-sufficiency.

sport dives, frequently make use of breathing gases other than normal air, and may include extended decompression. Most technical diving requires a much higher level of expertise on the part of the diver. Although technical divers frequently assert that they are not sport divers, they still are performing their dives for the purpose of recreation.

Surface-Supplied Diving

Surface-supplied diving is any type of diving done where the diver is provided with breathing gas from the surface via a long hose. On the surface, the hose may be connected to a low-pressure compressor which pumps air directly to the diver, or to a "bank" of high-pressure cylinders that provide either air or other gas mixtures.

Within the definition of surface-supplied diving there are several different modes of diving including "hookah" diving, surface-supplied air diving, surface-supplied mixed gas diving, bell bounce diving, and saturation diving.

Hookah Diving

Hookah diving is the simplest form of surface-supplied diving. A hookah unit usually consists of a small low-pressure air compressor which is connected to a low-pressure steel gas container called a "volume tank." Air is pumped from the compressor into the volume tank, which serves as a reservoir or short duration "reserve" supply. The volume tank also provides a method for cooling the air which allows any moisture to condense and collect in the bottom of the container where it can be periodically drained. The diver's breathing air hose connects directly to the volume tank.

At the end of the diver's air hose is a second stage scuba regulator. A few feet back from the end of the hose is a quick release snap hook so that the diver can attach the hose to a harness worn on his body. Thus, there is no direct tension on

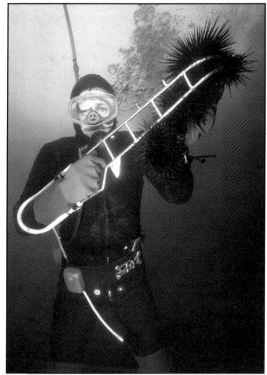

Fig. 2.7 Hookah gear is the most efficient diving equipment a commercial sea urchin diver can use underwater while collecting his catch.

the mouthpiece from the hose.

Divers in the following professions often use hookah:

- Seafood diving, such as divers who collect sea urchins
- Gold dredging in rivers and streams
- Divers who clean boat bottoms
- Treasure hunters

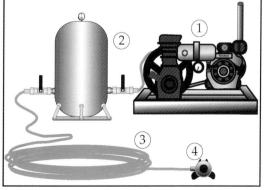

Fig. 2.8 A simple hookah system consists of a 1) compressor, 2) volume tank, 3) hose, and 4) scuba regulator second stage.

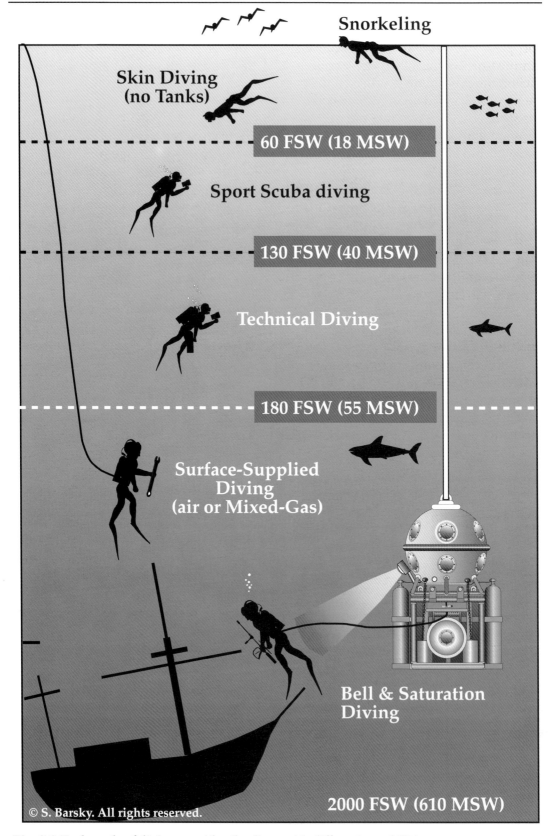

Snorkeling

Skin Diving
(no Tanks)

60 FSW (18 MSW)

Sport Scuba diving

130 FSW (40 MSW)

Technical Diving

180 FSW (55 MSW)

Surface-Supplied
Diving
(air or Mixed-Gas)

Bell & Saturation
Diving

2000 FSW (610 MSW)

© S. Barsky. All rights reserved.

Fig. 2.9 Each mode of diving provides the diver with different capabilities.

It is not unusual for divers using hookah gear to dive without any support personnel topside. In the event of a compressor failure, or if the boat drags anchor, the diver is on his own to sort out the problem. Accidents have occurred in this situation, for a variety of reasons.

A small number of recreational divers also use hookah gear. The type of system they use usually consists of a floating inner-tube or buoy which supports a small compressor. The hose is attached to a harness worn by the diver. The divers tow the float carrying the compressor as they swim along. These systems are limited by the small compressor used with them and cannot generally support divers much below 30 feet.

Umbilical Diving – Air

Umbilical diving usually refers to diving with a surface-supplied breathing gas source, but using a full-face mask or a diving helmet for the breathing system. The main reason for using the full-face mask or helmet is that it provides the

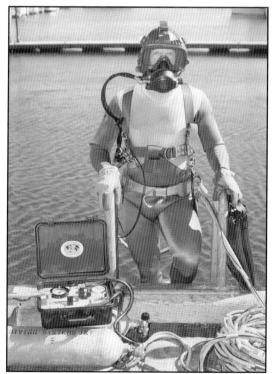

Fig. 2.10 Umbilical diving systems can be very simple.

diver with a means to communicate, as well as additional protection.

While a diver using hookah might dive alone, with no support personnel, a diver using a surface-supplied air system will have at least one person, and usually two, topside to assist him. On big jobs, there may be an entire crew of personnel topside, each performing a different task to assist the diver and helping to get the job done.

An umbilical diving system normally includes some type of breathing gas supply on the surface, an "umbilical" or diving hose, and a full-face mask or helmet. The umbilical usually consists of a breathing gas supply hose, a communications wire, and a depth sensing hose (pneumofathometer). It may also include a hot water hose, to warm the diver's suit.

The smallest diving crew that is considered to fall within acceptable safety standards for surface-supplied diving is a three-man crew. With a three man crew, one person dives, one person tends the hose for the diver in the water, and the third person is available to act as a "standby diver" or "safety diver," ready to go to the aid of the diver in the water should assistance be needed. When the first diver is done with the dive, the crew can rotate through each of the positions until the job is completed.

In the United States, surface-supplied air diving is normally conducted at depths down to 190 feet of sea water (FSW), although according to U.S. Coast Guard standards, dives with bottom times of 30 minutes or less may be conducted to 220 FSW. Industry standards, published by the Association of Diving Contractors International, do not set a time limit on air dives to 220 FSW, but from a practical standpoint, longer dives require extended decompression.

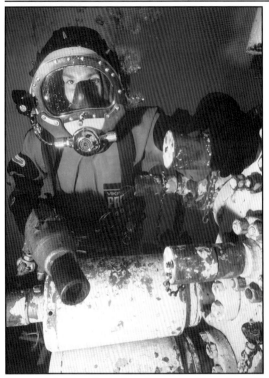

Fig. 2.11 The limit for deep air dives is 220 feet of sea water, but at this depth helium-oxygen mixtures are usually preferred.

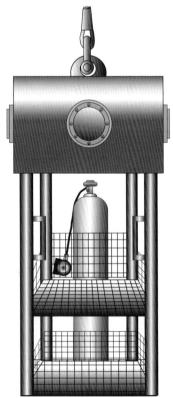

Fig. 2.12 An open bottom bell is mandatory for surface-supplied mixed gas dives.

Surface-Supplied Mixed Gas Diving

In surface-supplied mixed gas diving, the diver uses surface-supplied diving gear, but instead of breathing air at depth, the diver breathes a special gas mixture, that usually consists of helium and oxygen, or helium, oxygen and nitrogen (tri-mix). The purpose of this special gas mixture is to reduce the narcotic effects of nitrogen at depth, so the diver may function with a clear head.

The equipment for surface-supplied mixed gas diving is the same as that used in umbilical diving, but there are several important additions. The most obvious additions are the cylinders of specially mixed gas and the need for a helium-speech unscrambler. An "open bottom bell" is also considered essential for mixed-gas diving operations.

In the commercial field, surface-supplied mixed gas operations are conducted between depths of 150 and 300 feet of seawater. Beyond that depth, a closed diving bell is normally used. In some parts of the world, there are specific depth ranges at which certain types of gear must be used, according to government regulations.

Bell Bounce Diving

For deep, but relatively short-term dives, a bell "bounce" diving system is usually used. These systems are generally set up to accommodate no more than two divers at a time under pressure. Bounce dives are generally made to depths not over 500 feet.

The crew for a bell bounce diving operation may be as small as six people, with two divers in the bell, and four crewmembers topside.

Saturation Diving

The concept behind saturation diving is very simple. While decompression is always dependent on the diver's depth, once a diver has been under pressure continuously for 24 hours his decompres-

Band mask drawing © Kirby Morgan Dive Systems, Inc. All rights reserved.

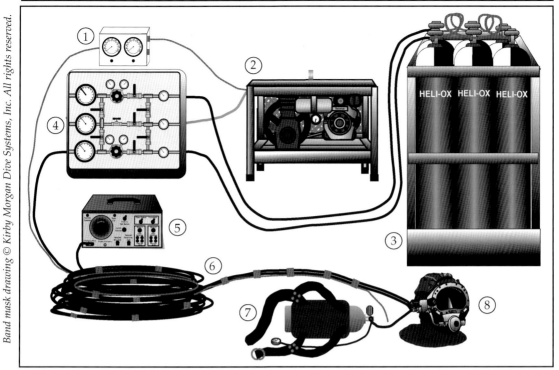

Fig. 2.13 Life support gear for a basic mixed gas system would include the following gear: 1) Pneumofathometer panel, 2) low pressure air compressor, 3) Helium-oxygen gas cylinders, 4) Mixed gas control panel, 5) Helium speech unscrambler, 6) Umbilical, 7) Bailout bottle and harness, and 8) Full-face mask or helmet.

sion from that depth remains the same whether he has been under pressure for one day or 10 days.

After the first 24-hour period under pressure the diver's body is said to be completely saturated with inert gas for that specific depth. Once this happens, decompression from the dive takes roughly one day for every 100 feet of depth. For example, decompression from a 500 foot saturation dive would take somewhere between five and six days (or 5 X 100, plus a bit more). Different commercial diving companies use proprietary decompression tables with varying decompression schedules. Some tables are much "faster" than others, but the risk of decompression sickness may also be higher.

Saturation diving is an extremely efficient way to work underwater if the job will be deep and/or of long duration. While saturated at a particular depth, within certain limits, the diver can do downward "excursions" and upward "excursions" without changing the saturation storage depth.

On large projects, there may be as many as six divers living in the saturation complex topside, rotating in and out of the diving bell for their shift underwater. Each team of divers has approximately 24 hours off to eat, sleep, and get rested before their next dive.

Each bell run usually lasts for anywhere from ten to twelve hours, with each diver spending about four hours in the water. An experienced topside crew can "turn the bell around" in about an hour from the time the bell hits the deck until it is back in the water on its way to the bottom.

Since the diving on a saturation system goes on around the clock, there will normally be two complete topside crews, each working a twelve-hour shift, to sup-

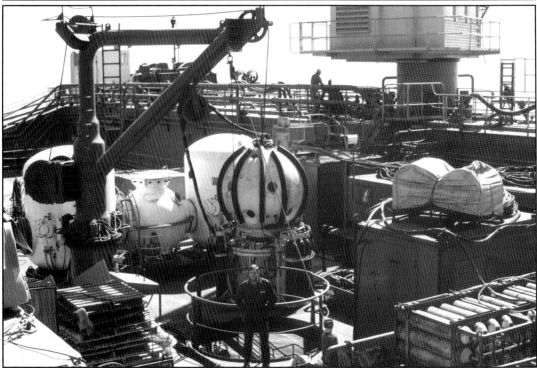

Fig. 2.14 Both bell bounce dives and saturation dives could be made with the system shown here. This system was installed on a drill rig in the North Sea. The diving bell is the sphere in the center of the photo and the two white vertical chambers and spherical entrance lock are behind the bell. In the right foreground are racks of mixed gas.

port the divers in the system. The crew might be comprised of the following:

Day shift	Night shift
Supervisor	Supervisor
Lead diver	Lead diver
(topside)	(topside)
Diver	Diver
Tenders (2 ea.)	Tenders (2 ea.)
Life support tech	Life support tech

6 additional divers in saturation

On some jobs, the deck crew may even be conducting shallow air dives at the same time as the bell is in the water, but the crew will need to be much larger.

Case History – Professional Seafood Diver

Commercial sea urchin diving has been an important fishery in many states including Alaska, California, Maine, Oregon, and Washington. Divers typically work out of small, fast boats, with one or two divers per boat and at most, one tender to assist the diver.

In some states, the divers use hookah gear to provide their air supply, with a small gasoline or diesel driven compressor topside. Floating diving hose is generally preferred by these divers to avoid entanglement with rocks and marine growth. The hose floats on the water to a point on the surface close to the diver and then usually runs at a diagonal down to the diver where it is clipped off to his chest.

Numerous accidents have occurred due to the failure of these divers to utilize the code alpha flag or the sport diving flag, or where boat operators have failed to recognize the meaning of these flags, or the type of dive operation being conducted. In these cases, the diver's hose is usually snagged by the boat and either the hose is severed or the diver is dragged off the bottom.

In at least one incident where the diver's hose was severed, the diver was killed, by drowning. In incidents where the divers have been dragged off the bottom, they may consequently suffer from decompression sickness. Proving or disproving a case of decompression sickness may be difficult.

One of the more interesting cases that occurred involved a sport diving group that was operating an inflatable near a popular diving area. En route to the dive site, they passed several urchin diving boats where the tenders aboard the boat waived them off in a particular direction.

As they passed the last boat, the person on board gave no indication they had a diver in the water so the group in the inflatable continued on their intended heading. In addition, the boat was not displaying any day shapes or flying either the alpha flag or the sport diving flag. Unbeknownst to the skipper of the inflatable, they had snagged the hose of the urchin diver working off the boat and jerked him off the bottom.

A confrontation ensued between the urchin diver and the inflatable operator and a lawsuit was filed. The case was tried in admiralty court.

The diver not only alleged that he suffered decompression sickness, but also that he was injured as he twisted around in the water as he attempted to control his hose. The court decided the case in favor of the diver, although it disallowed his claims of decompression sickness and gave him an award based upon the physical injuries he claimed occurred as a result of twisting around to try to release his hose.

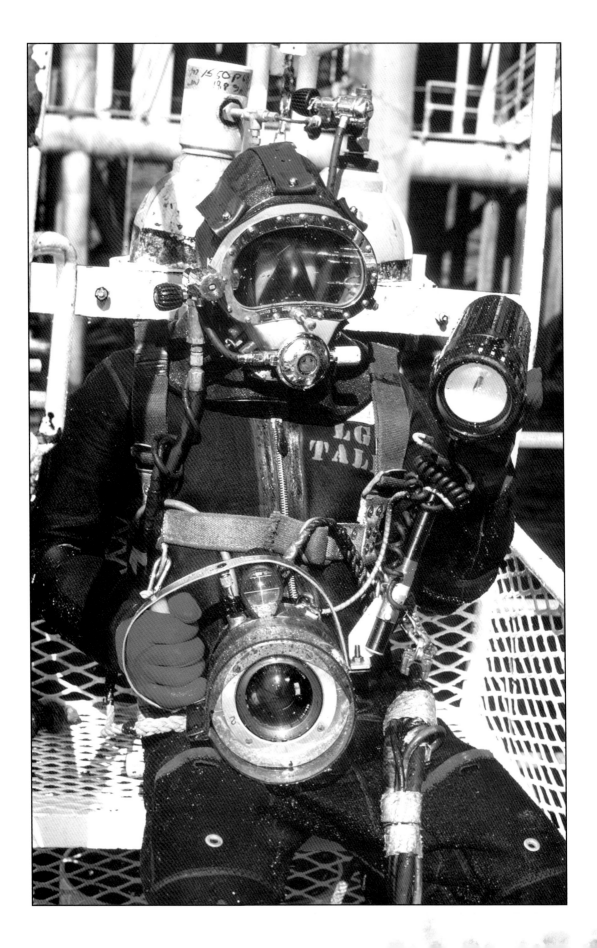

Chapter 3
Types of Diving Equipment

The majority of diving equipment manufactured today is high quality and extremely reliable. In this section we'll look at different types of dive gear, how they are used, and what role they may play in an accident. While almost any piece of gear can fail and cause difficulty for a person underwater, divers are routinely trained to deal with gear failures. A properly trained diver should be capable of dealing with minor gear problems. However, even minor gear failures can cause inexperienced divers to panic, leading to accidents.

The same diving equipment used by recreational divers may also be used by scientific divers, commercial divers, and law enforcement divers. Although commercial divers tend to prefer equipment that is more heavy duty, a sport diver, a diving scientist, and a commercial diver could all conceivably use the same type of fins or wear the same type of wetsuit. On the other hand, items such as commercial diving helmets tend to be used only by professional and commercial divers.

Most diving equipment in the United States is manufactured to a high standard, but there is no government or industry standard that covers all gear manufactured in the U.S. The U.S. Navy has set standards for breathing apparatus for military use, and regulators sold into the civilian market are frequently evaluated against this standard.

Equipment sold in Europe must meet standards set in Europe and carry the mark "CE," and many U.S. manufacturers design and test their gear to meet these standards. Equipment with the "CE" mark may be sold into any country participating in the European Economic Community.

Diver Worn Equipment vs. Support Equipment

In recreational diving, almost all of the equipment used for diving, is worn or

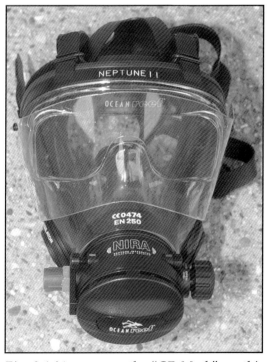

Fig. 3.1 You can see the "CE Mark" on this full-face mask just above the word NIRA on the regulator.

carried by the diver himself.

In professional and commercial diving, there may be a great deal of equipment used to support the diving operation that is not worn by the diver. These items may include breathing gas control manifolds, diving hoses, diving bells, decompression chambers, and similar items.

Diver Worn Equipment
Face Masks

Face masks are rarely defective, but they are frequently abused by divers. Even if a mask fails underwater, one of the first skills that all divers are taught is how to breathe without a mask underwater. The loss or failure of a mask should not be a cause for panic for the properly trained diver. Face masks used for scuba diving generally cover the eyes and nose, but not the mouth. There is a different type of mask, known as a "full-face mask" (that covers the mouth as well) that can also be used with scuba equipment, that will be discussed later in this chapter.

Mask failures can occur in three different ways. The most common problem with face masks is a broken head strap. Even then, the diver can hold the mask to his face to return to the surface. If the mask is completely lost, it is still possible to see underwater, although the diver's vision will be blurry. It is not uncommon for a diver whose mask is flooded or lost

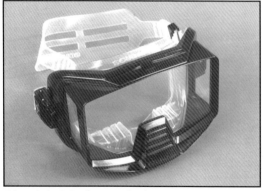

Fig. 3.2 Masks made by reputable diving equipment manufacturers use tempered glass for the lens.

to accidentally inhale water through the nose. This can lead to coughing which can cause a diver to panic, or drop his regulator from his mouth, causing further problems.

It is unusual for a diver to break the lens of his mask underwater, but it can happen if conditions are rough. Most people will naturally extend their arms ahead of them if they are being carried towards a rock or wreckage by wave action in an instinctive move to protect their face and head. Good quality face masks are made with tempered glass which will not shatter in the event of impact, but forms "pebbles" like automotive glass. Poor quality masks may use ordinary glass or cheap plastic. If you are investigating an accident and find broken shards of glass in the mask it's a reasonable conclusion that the mask was not made by a reputable diving equipment manufacturer.

Masks can also fail if the frame for the lens is damaged or the flexible skirt that seals against the face is torn. Most masks today are manufactured either from hypoallergenic silicone or other high quality rubber and these types of failures are uncommon. A mask frame or seal is rarely damaged during the course of a dive and any failure that occurred in storage or en route to the dive site is usually obvious to the user prior to diving.

Snorkels

A snorkel is a simple breathing tube with a mouthpiece on one end. They are used by skin divers or breath-hold divers as their breathing apparatus. The snorkel allows the skin diver to keep his face in the water and observe the underwater world through his mask while resting on the surface and breathing through the snorkel. Snorkels are used by scuba divers for swimming on the surface to and from the dive site to conserve the air in their scuba cylinders. However, some divers today routinely do their surface swimming on their back, so the absence

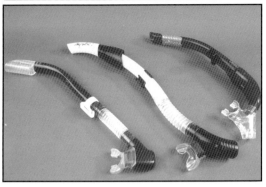

Fig. 3.3 Snorkels are used for swimming on the surface to conserve scuba air.

Fins

Fins are designed to move the diver through the water quickly, and there are hundreds of different fin designs. Fins for snorkeling in warm water usually include a foot pocket to attach the fin to the foot, but most other types of diving fins usually use a strap to hold the fin on the foot. Rubber foot pockets eventually wear out or rot as do fin straps.

Most fin straps are either rubber or cloth. The straps are attached to the fins usually by mounting hardware made from chromed brass, stainless steel, or plastic. Mounting hardware can fail too, although this is less common. When mounting hardware fails it is usually due to some type of physical damage.

When a fin pocket or strap fails it can be difficult for a person wearing a thick diving suit to swim effectively, particularly if they are wearing any type of breathing apparatus with straps that go over the shoulders. Both the suit and the straps of the breathing apparatus will restrict arm movement. A person who is snorkeling in warm water, wearing nothing more than a bathing suit doesn't face the same problem, so the loss of a fin in this situation is usually not as serious.

of a snorkel may not be indicative of a problem.

Many snorkels today are equipped with special valves to prevent water from reaching the diver's mouthpiece and to make it easier to clear any water that has found its way into the snorkel. The failure of these valves could lead a diver who was dependent on their snorkel for surface swimming to have a problem, but this would be unusual. Even divers who routinely use their snorkels will frequently swim on their backs.

It would be unusual for a snorkel to be a major contributing factor in a diving accident.

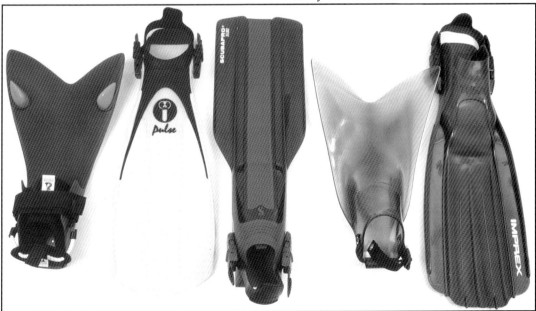

Fig. 3.4 The loss of a fin makes it difficult for a scuba diver to move through the water.

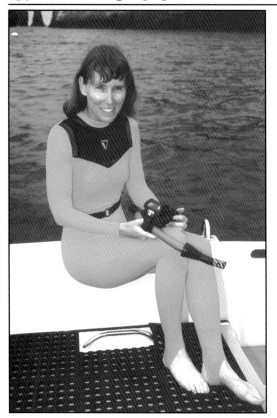

Fig. 3.5 Lycra® dive skins are worn for sun and abrasion protection in tropical waters.

Even without fins, a diver should be able to establish positive buoyancy and float on the surface. In most cases, once the diver is floating on the surface, danger is greatly reduced. The loss of a fin becomes more critical in situations where a scuba diver must swim to escape some type of hazardous situation, such as to exit from a cave, to avoid being thrown onto rocks by wave action, or to avoid boat traffic on the surface.

Thermal Protection

Divers use four major different types of suits. Suit selection by sport divers is usually dependent on the water temperature, the type of diving activity that the diver enjoys, and the diver's personal budget.

Suit selection by commercial divers is dependent on water temperature and budget, too, but frequently the job

at hand will dictate the type of suit that should be worn. Both sport and working divers make inappropriate choices in thermal protection and their use and these mistakes can lead to fatalities. Both sport and commercial divers use wetsuits and dry suits, however, commercial divers also use a type of protection known as a "hot water suit."

Dive Skins

"Dive skins" are a type of body suit worn for diving that usually offer little or no thermal protection, but do provide protection from sunburn, jellyfish, and abrasion. Dive skins may be made from a variety of different materials including Lycra® and other synthetics. These suits are typically worn only for recreational diving in the tropics.

Wetsuits

Wetsuits are made from foam neoprene rubber. In theory, the wetsuit keeps the diver warm by allowing a thin layer of water to enter the suit. This water is warmed by the diver's body. If the suit fits well and the water is not too cold, wetsuits are a cost effective method of thermal protection for short duration dives. Sport, professional, and commercial divers all may use wetsuits.

A wetsuit can be torn or its zipper can fail and the suit will still provide some degree of thermal protection. However, in waters colder than 65 degrees F or for long duration dives, wetsuits may not provide adequate thermal protection.

Hypothermia (chilling of the body core) is probably a bigger factor in diving accidents than most people realize. As the diver's core temperature drops, the diver's ability to think clearly drops and manual dexterity decreases. On extended dives, hypothermia can occur even in relatively warm water.

As a diver becomes increasingly uncomfortable due to the cold, he may make judgement errors in attempts to avoid discomfort. For example, divers have been known to skip precautionary, or actual, decompression stops in an effort to get out of the water.

Wetsuits provide no protection for commercial divers working in polluted water, as any contaminants will enter the suit through the zipper, wrists, neck, and ankles. Many chemicals will destroy wetsuit material.

It is impossible for a dive store to stock every size of rental wetsuit and it is not uncommon for divers in training to end up using rental suits that are either too tight or too loose. In either case, the suit can contribute to a diver's discomfort. A suit that is too loose on a thin or small diver can contribute to hypothermia. A suit that is too tight on a large or overweight diver can cause the diver to overheat topside and may restrict the diver's ability to breathe comfortably, especially in situations of high stress, such as making an entry through surf. This can lead to feelings of anxiety which can end in panic.

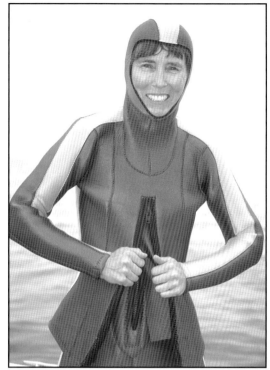

Fig. 3.6 Wetsuits provide reasonable thermal protection for water temperatures down to about 65 degrees F.

Dry Suits

Dry suits offer better thermal protection in cold water than wetsuits, but dry suits are more expensive to purchase, and maintain. They also require additional training for their use. For these reasons, dry suits are seen less commonly in most areas than wetsuits. Without proper training, or if the diver fails to maintain the suit properly, there is potential for a dry suit accident.

Dry suits are made from a variety of materials including foam neoprene, crushed neoprene, polyurethane, tri-laminate materials, and vulcanized rubber. The suit is constructed using special techniques to make the seams waterproof.

Unlike a wetsuit, a dry suit is made to completely seal the water out of the suit. This is achieved by using a waterproof zipper to allow the diver to enter the suit, and special seals at the wrists and neck.

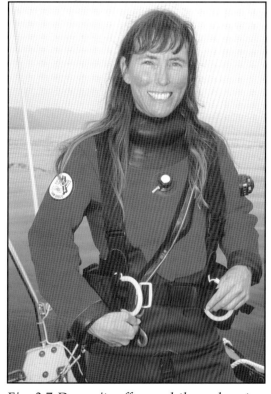

Fig. 3.7 Dry suits offer good thermal protection for the coldest of water temperatures.

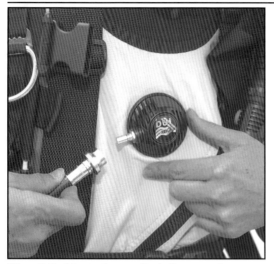

Fig. 3.8 Most dry suit inflator valves are located in the center of the chest on the suit. They use low-pressure air from the diver's tank.

There is an inflator valve (usually located on the chest) to add air to the suit, and an exhaust valve (usually located on the left arm) to vent air from the suit. Any of these components can fail to function properly. This type of problem can be compounded if the diver has not received adequate training to dive the suit.

Most dry suits are not designed to provide any insulation by themselves. Thermal underwear must be worn under the suit to capture the diver's body heat. The diver stays warm because the heat from his body is trapped inside the air layer in the dry suit underwear.

The diver adds air to the dry suit to provide insulation, to prevent the suit from "squeezing" his body, and to control buoyancy. If the diver does not add any air to the suit, it will start to pinch his body as he descends. In addition, as the diver descends, if no air is added to the suit, the diver will become increasingly heavy as the air already inside the suit compresses. To offset the effects of pressure, the diver must add small amounts of air to the suit. Dry suits are considered passive insulation and are most effective for dives where air is the breathing medium.

Because the diver adds and vents air from the suit itself during the dive, proper dry suit training is essential. Without proper training, divers may add too much weight to their weight belts while using a dry suit, in a mistaken attempt to control buoyancy. With excess weight added, it becomes difficult to control the large bubble of air in the suit, especially if the diver inverts and is untrained in how to recover to an upright position. Other dry suit accidents have involved zippers that have failed, defective or damaged valves, and damaged or improperly adjusted seals.

Dry suit valves that have been improperly maintained can become jammed open or closed. An exhaust valve that is jammed open can allow all of the air in the suit to escape and cause the suit to flood. When an exhaust valve is jammed closed, there is no way to vent air from the valve and the suit can over-inflate unless the diver vents air through the neck seal or wrist seal.

The main types of adverse events that occur with dry suits involve a loss of buoyancy control. In one set of circum-

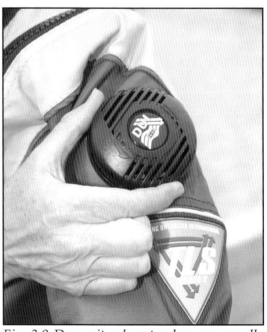

Fig. 3.9 Dry suit exhaust valves are usually located on the diver's left upper arm.

stances, the diver becomes too buoyant and may rise uncontrollably to the surface. In this setting, a lung over-pressure injury or decompression sickness may occur. If the zipper on the suit fails, or the suit is torn, or a valve is damaged, it may be difficult for the diver to maintain neutral buoyancy underwater or positive buoyancy at the surface.

If an inflator valve is stuck open, air will continually fill the suit, unless the diver disconnects the air supply hose. If the inflator is jammed shut, which is quite uncommon, there is no way to add air to the suit.

Although both sport and commercial divers wear dry suits, the types of suits worn by commercial divers tend to be heavier duty. Working divers use dry suits for dives in polluted water to protect their bodies from contaminants. Not only is the material thicker on most suits used for commercial diving, but the zipper is also usually of a much more robust design.

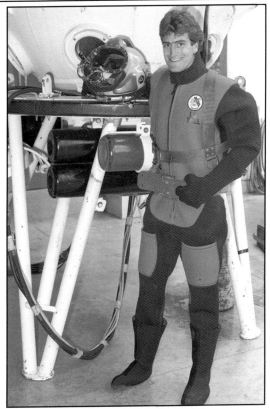

Fig. 3.10 Hot water suits are used for commercial diving, especially on dives where the diver is breathing helium-oxygen gas mixtures.

Hot Water Suits

A hot water suit is a large, loose fitting diving suit, that is equipped with perforated hoses that run inside the suit down each arm and leg, as well as down the front and back of the torso. A special valve, which connects to these tubes, is located at the waist of the suit, and provides a connection for the hot water hose from the surface. The valve has two positions, "on" or "by-pass," which directs the water away from the suit.

The suit itself is usually made from a dense, crushed neoprene material with a heavy-duty nylon coating on the outside of the suit. The material has little or no buoyancy.

When hot water enters the suit, it circulates around the diver and flows out through the wrists, ankle, and neck opening of the suit. Without a continuous flow of hot water, the diver would chill very quickly. Special hot water suits are available with non-return valves to prevent the loss of the hot water in the suit and rapid chilling of the diver in the event of a hot water system failure.

Special hot water machines located topside generate the hot water that is supplied to the diver. These machines may be diesel or electrically operated. On a barge equipped with a steam system, it's also possible to generate hot water in this way.

Hot water suits are an extremely efficient way to keep a diver warm under demanding conditions. They are considered essential for deep diving, especially when the diver is breathing helium, because of helium's high "thermal conductivity." Heat loss from the lungs is very high for divers at great depths. Without the hot water suit, deep saturation diving would be essentially impossible due to the high thermal demands of this type of diving, where active heating of the diver and his inspired gas is vital.

Aside from the failure of the hot water system, there have also been events when the diver has been scalded because the water supplied by the hot water system was too warm. In addition, there have been incidents where the hot water system intake has picked up jellyfish floating at the surface and pumped the stinging tentacles down inside the diver's suit.

Weight Belts and Weight Systems

Weight belts are worn to offset the buoyancy of a wetsuit, dry suit, or other pieces of equipment. Belts may be made from nylon webbing, rubber, or plastic. The buckles are usually made from either plastic or stainless steel.

Diving weights are available either as solid weights in increments from two through ten pounds, or as shot filled bags. Solid weights are slotted and slip onto the belt, while shot pouches must be used with a belt designed with compartments to hold them.

For recreational diving, the belt buckles are designed to have a quick release mechanism so that the weights may be ditched in an emergency and the buckle may be activated with one hand. For commercial diving, quick release buckles are considered undesirable, because of the possibility that the belt may come off accidentally when the diver has a decom-

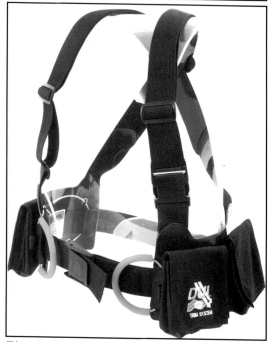

Fig. 3.12 Recreational divers may use a weight harness like this one that distributes the weight across the diver's shoulders.

pression obligation. Ditching a weight belt designed for commercial diving use is normally a two-handed operation.

There are also weight harnesses that are designed for recreational diving as well as those designed for commercial diving. Weight harnesses have shoulder straps that criss-cross over the diver's back, although the weights themselves still are attached to a belt around the diver's waist. The purpose of the weight harness is to distribute and support the weight across the diver's shoulders rather than making the diver's lower back support the load.

By themselves, weight belts rarely cause any type of accident, other than when a belt falls on a diver's foot. However, a common finding in accident investigations is the failure of a diver to either ditch his weight belt or inflate his buoyancy compensator in an emergency situation.

In rare circumstances, a weight belt may be trapped between a buoyancy compensator and the diver's back or hang

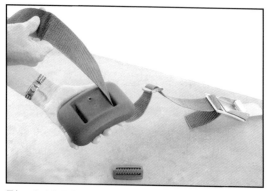

Fig. 3.11 Diving weights are made from lead. They may be coated with plastic or bare, or sold as shot filled bags.

up on a knife mounted on the diver's leg. If the buoyancy compensator is equipped with a crotch strap, it's also possible for the diver to mistakenly fasten the strap over the belt, making it impossible to drop the belt.

Buoyancy Compensators

Buoyancy compensators are the devices that sport divers wear to control their flotation. They may also be referred to as a "BC" or BCD (buoyancy compensator device).

These devices incorporate an inflatable bladder and are commonly inflated with low-pressure air from the scuba cylinder. The components of the buoyancy compensator include the following:

• An inflatable bladder – The bladder may be mounted behind the diver's back or may form a vest that surrounds the diver's torso.

• A corrugated hose allowing air to flow into the bladder – The hose is generally located on the left side of the bladder and attaches at or close to shoulder level. In the diving industry, manufacturers typically refer to this hose as an "airway."

• An overinflation valve – This is a one-way valve designed to relieve pressure in the buoyancy compensator in the event the diver fails to vent the pressure manually. The primary function of the overinflation valve is to prevent the inflatable bladder from rupturing. This type of valve may also be referred to as a relief valve.

• An inflator mechanism – This is a device designed to put air into the buoyancy compensator. Most inflator mechanisms today allow the diver to add air manually, by placing his mouth on the mechanism, pushing a button and blowing air into the BC or by pushing a button which allows air to enter the buoyancy compensator via a hose connected to the

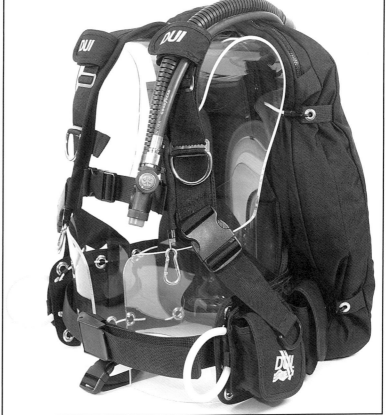

Fig. 3.13 There are many different designs of buoyancy compensators.

first stage of the diver's regulator. These devices are also referred to as "power inflators." Some power inflators are designed to serve a secondary function as emergency breathing regulators. The inflator also usually includes a button to vent air from the buoyancy compensator.

• Remote exhaust – The remote exhaust is a redundant exhaust mechanism that allows the diver to vent air from the buoyancy compensator by pulling down on the corrugated inflator hose, rather than lifting the hose and inflator mechanism overhead to vent. Inside the corrugated hose is a stainless steel wire that connects to the second exhaust mechanism which is mounted where the corrugated hose attaches to the bladder. The remote exhaust is usually an option on most buoyancy compensators.

• Tank bands – Most buoyancy compensators are designed to also carry the diver's tank (air supply). The tank bands are usually made from heavy duty webbing, use a plastic buckle to fasten them, and have Velcro® to further secure them. There is only one proper method for threading the tank buckle and if this strap is improperly threaded the tank can fall out of the pack. Tanks have fallen and hit other divers aboard dive boats and tanks have come loose underwater.

• Shoulder and waist straps – The shoulder and waist straps secure the buoyancy compensator to the diver's body. Most shoulder straps are adjustable.

Diving accidents can occur when divers are unable to control their buoyancy properly. It is, of course, possible for a power inflator to be defective. It is also possible, for power inflators to leak air into the buoyancy compensator, giving the diver unwanted buoyancy.

Buoyancy compensators can and do develop leaks if they are improperly maintained or the device has seen prolonged or severe service. However, even a leaking buoyancy compensator will usually hold more than enough air to provide the diver with positive buoyancy. While buoyancy compensator bladders can be defective, it is rare for one to spontaneously fail.

Scuba Cylinders and Valves

Scuba cylinders are made from primarily one of two materials, aluminum or chrome molybdenum steel. Although other materials have been tested, these are the two most common materials used.

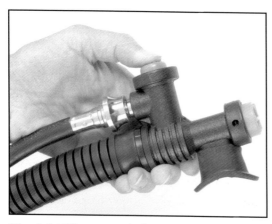
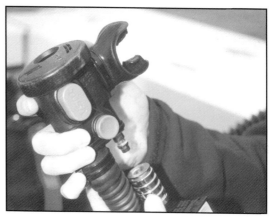

Fig. 3.14 The power inflator receives low-pressure air from the first stage of the diver's regulator. The model on the left only provides inflation for the buoyancy compensator. The model on the right also performs as an emergency breathing regulator.

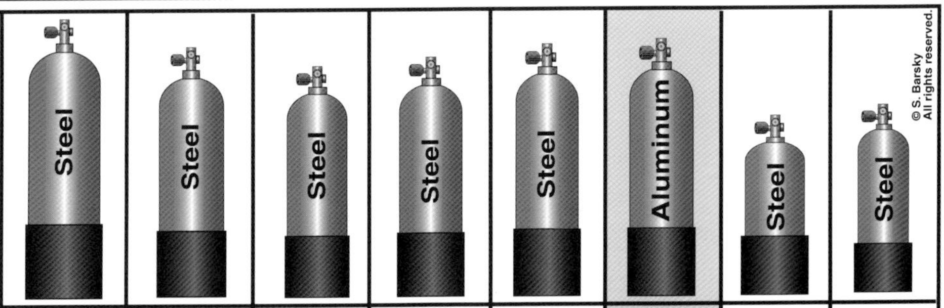

Relative Cylinder Sizes & Volumes listed by weight Imperial Version	Steel	Steel	Steel	Steel	Steel	Aluminum	Steel	Steel
Volume	125 cu. ft.	112 cu. ft.	98 cu. ft.	100 cu. ft.	85 cu. ft.	80 cu. ft.	80 cu. ft.	66 cu. ft.
Length	29"	26"	24"	25.2"	26"	27"	21"	21"
Diameter	8"	8"	8"	7.3"	7"	7.25"	7.3"	7"
Weight	45 lb.	41 lb.	38 lb.	36 lb.	31 lb.	31 lb.	31 lb.	25 lb.
Working Pressure	2640 p.s.i.	2640 p.s.i.	2640 p.s.i.	3500 p.s.i.	3500 p.s.i.	3000 p.s.i.	3500 p.s.i.	2640p.s.i.
Buoyancy Full	-9.5 lb.	-8 lb.	-7.73 lb.	-11.5 lb.	-6.7 lb.	-1.4 lb.	-10.9 lb.	- 5 lb.
Buoyancy Empty	neutral	-1 lb.	neutral	-5 lb.	neutral	+4.4 lb.	-4 lb.	-1.67 lb.

© S. Barsky. All rights reserved.

Fig. 3.15 Scuba tanks are made from different materials and come in a variety of sizes. Each one has its own buoyancy characteristics. There are more varieties than what is shown here.

Each different size of scuba cylinder has its own buoyancy characteristics, depending on the dimensions of the cylinder, its internal volume, and the material used to manufacture it. Whenever a diver uses a different scuba cylinder, a procedure known as a "buoyancy check" is essential to verify that the diver is properly weighted for the combination of gear he is wearing. A chart of the weights, sizes, and buoyancy characteristics of some common scuba cylinders is shown at the top of this page.

Although scuba cylinders rarely contribute to in-water diving accidents, there have been numerous cylinder failures on dry land that have occurred during the filling of cylinders. When a cylinder explodes, the results can be fatal.

Both steel and aluminum cylinders are subject to corrosion. Corrosion is usually more of a problem internally than it is externally, and is probably the most common form of failure in steel cylinders. Metal fatigue, undetected flaws, and cracks are problems that occur more com-

monly with aluminum cylinders.

The valves that control the air flow in and out of scuba cylinders tend to be highly reliable. Most of the valves used on modern scuba cylinders tend to be simple on and off valves. These are commonly referred to as "K" valves.

Older scuba cylinders were sometimes equipped with valves that were designed to provide a reserve supply of air, commonly referred to as "J" valves. These valves included a spring loaded mechanism that was set at a pressure anywhere between 300 and 500 p.s.i. When the air pressure in the cylinder dropped to this pressure, the reserve valve would start to close, gradually restricting the air supply to the diver, making it harder to breathe. The diver could reach back and activate a lever or rod on the side of the tank and open the reserve to gain access to the remaining air supply. This valve action was supposed to signal the diver that it was time to ascend. This type of valve is rarely encountered today.

Accidents occurred with this older

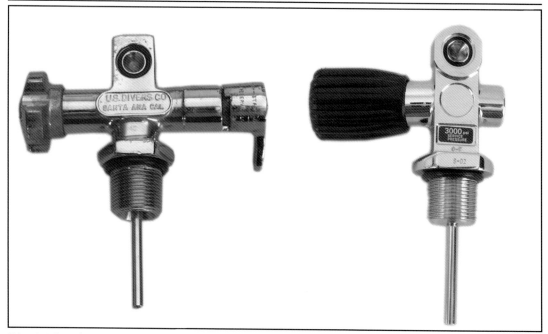

Fig. 3.16 and 3.17 "J" valves (like the valve on the left) were popular in the early days of diving, but are rarely seen in use today. This valve has a reserve function.

The "K" valve (shown on the right) is the primary valve in use today for sport diving. This valve is designed to be used with a regulator with a yoke connection that slips over the valve. This valve has no reserve function.

valve design because if the valve caught on anything or bumped anything underwater, the air supply would bypass the reserve, and the diver could breathe all the air in the tank without experiencing any restriction until the air supply was almost gone. When this happened, and the diver then attempted to access the reserve, he would suddenly find himself with no additional air. Some divers panicked when this occurred, sometimes with disastrous results.

Although it is rare to see a "J" valve anymore, there are still some in use. Since most divers are not trained to use a "J" valve today, this type of valve could be a contributing factor in an accident.

Scuba cylinder valves are designated by the amount of pressure they are designed to handle. For tank pressures of 3000 p.s.i. or less, most cylinders will be equipped with a traditional "yoke" design, where the first stage of the regulator slips over the outside of the valve and a large "set screw" is tightened to secure

the regulator to the valve. The tank valve has a machined groove that contains an o-ring where the regulator connects to the valve.

Although scuba cylinder valves themselves rarely play a role in diving accidents, more than one fatality has occurred when a diver used a tank with the valve only minimally opened. Upon reaching depth, the minimally opened valve made the diver believe there was no air. Panic then ensued, sometimes resulting in a fatal accident.

Scuba cylinders that are designed for tank pressures above 3000 p.s.i. are normally equipped with a "DIN" valve. DIN is a German abbreviation which stands for Deutsche Industrie fuer Normeng. This is a European gas fitting standard that is also popular in the U.S.

The DIN valve uses a "captured o-ring system." On a DIN valve, the regulator actually screws into threads inside the tank valve. The DIN system is generally considered to be a safer system because there is less chance of the o-ring "escaping" from the valve, causing the diver to lose his air supply through leakage.

All modern scuba valves are equipped with an internal "snorkel" that extends into the cylinder, designed to prevent any foreign matter that might be inside the tank from blocking the airflow through the valve should the diver invert. The snorkel usually extends three to four inches beyond the bottom of the valve body. The theory behind the valve snorkel is that if the diver turns upside down and there is foreign matter inside the tank, the open end of the snorkel will be above any foreign matter

Regulators

Scuba regulators are designed to take the high-pressure air in the scuba cylinder and reduce the pressure to the exact pressure surrounding the diver. When the diver inhales, the regulator supplies air as he "demands" it. When inhalation stops air flow ceases. As the diver exhales, the air is released from the regulator through an exhaust valve. This type of equipment is known as "open-circuit" scuba gear.

The modern single hose regulator is divided into two "stages." The first stage

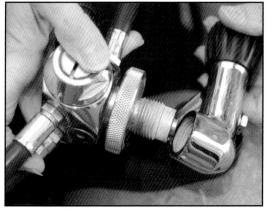

Fig. 3.18 DIN regulators actually thread into the tank valve.

attaches to the scuba cylinder at the valve and reduces the pressure in the tank to an intermediate pressure of approximately 140 p.s.i. over the surrounding pressure. A low-pressure hose connects the first stage to the second stage through a threaded opening known as a "low-pressure port."

The first stage may be designed to connect to the tank with either a yoke or a DIN fitting. Some regulators are shipped with an adapter that allows them to be used with either type of system.

Most modern regulators have at least three low-pressure ports and sometimes

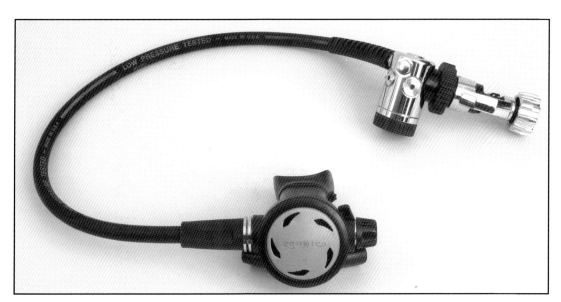

Fig. 3.19 Scuba regulators provide air to the diver only when he inhales through the mouthpiece.

more. Low-pressure ports are usually, but not always, identified by the letters "L.P." that are marked on the first stage. Other hoses that connect to the low-pressure ports might include:

• A low-pressure hose for the power inflator for the buoyancy compensator
• A low-pressure hose for the dry suit inflator
• An additional second stage used to supply emergency breathing air to another diver.

This is usually referred to as either a "safe-second" or an "octopus rig."
• A low-pressure hose to supply air to an air powered tool

There are also usually at least two "high-pressure ports." High-pressure ports are normally identified by the letters "H.P." The sole purpose of the high-pressure port is to provide a connection for a pressure sensing device, usually a simple gauge, to allow the diver to know the amount of air pressure remaining in his tank. The reason most regulators have more than one high-pressure port is to allow the diver to route the high-pressure hose over whichever shoulder he prefers.

Serious injuries have occurred when divers have connected low-pressure hoses to high-pressure ports. The low-pressure hose may explode, throwing pieces of hose and hose fittings great distances with tremendous force. Most regulators today use different size threads on the low-pressure and high-pressure ports to prevent this type of accident from happening.

Both low-pressure hoses and high-pressure hoses thread into the first stage and seal with small rubber o-rings. When these o-rings fail, the diver can lose a significant amount of breathing gas.

Low-pressure and high-pressure hoses can fail during routine use. Both types of failure will lead to a loss of air from the scuba cylinder.

The second stage of the regulator reduces the intermediate air pressure to the exact surrounding pressure, wherever the diver happens to be. This is also known as the "ambient pressure." The mouthpiece through which the diver inhales is part of the second stage.

Ideally, the regulator should provide this air with a minimum of resistance when the diver inhales. Likewise, the regulator should also allow the diver to exhale with as little resistance as possible.

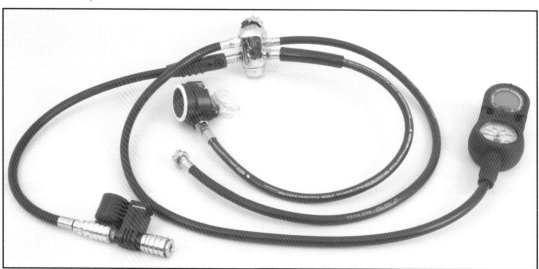

Fig. 3.20 This regulator has been configured for dry suit diving. It includes an inflator hose for the suit, another one for the buoyancy compensator, and a submersible pressure gauge.

The standards for regulator performance are well established and widely known throughout the diving industry. For this reason, there are very few regulators on the market today that do not offer high performance. Most modern regulators make it easy for the diver to breathe underwater.

Scuba regulators today are quite reliable, even when they have been improperly maintained and serviced. It is extremely rare for a regulator to "fail" and cause a diving accident.

There are only two failure modes for a regulator. The regulator can stop delivering air, which is rare, or the regulator can go into "free-flow" mode, where it flows air continuously, and exhausts the diver's air supply.

There are a number of factors that could cause a regulator to stop delivering air. These would include a blockage of internal orifices, a failure of the diaphragm that senses water pressure, or a hose failure. More commonly, a regulator might free-flow due to improper maintenance, sand entering the mouthpiece, low temperatures, or other causes.

The rubber parts of regulators are usually more prone to failure than the metal parts. Rubber parts rot and wear out due to exposure to sun, ozone from smog, chemicals in the water, and other causes. Regulators have external rubber parts that are visible, such as hoses, mouthpieces, exhaust shrouds or "Tees", and covers. These external rubber parts should always be carefully examined during any dive accident investigation.

The internal rubber parts of regulators include exhaust valves, sealing o-rings, and diaphragms. These parts are also subject to wear.

Regulators that are not properly maintained may have higher breathing resistance than normal. This increased resistance could be a contributing factor to a diving accident, particularly for a diver who is out of shape.

Most modern regulators breathe so easily that the diver can use the entire contents of the tank without noticing any significant increase in breathing resistance.

Instruments

During any dive accident investigation, it is essential for the investigator to carefully examine any instruments carried by the diver. These devices may provide extremely important clues as to what took place.

Submersible Pressure Gauge

The submersible pressure gauge is a device designed to continuously measure the pressure in the diver's tank while he is underwater. These gauges are subjected to great abuse and are frequently not precisely accurate. They are subject to flooding and once salt water enters the mechanism it is not uncommon for them

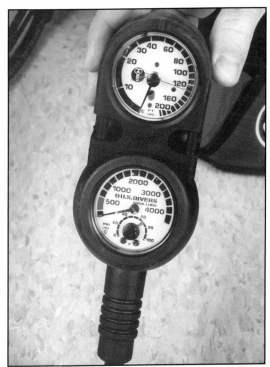

Fig. 3.21 Gauge consoles like this one that include a submersible pressure gauge (bottom) and depth gauge (top) are common.

to fail to register pressure accurately.

Diving accidents have occurred when divers have not realized that the submersible pressure gauge they were using was not functioning properly. The needle on the gauge can "freeze" at a low-pressure, but still be above zero, so that the diver thinks air is remaining in the tank when in fact there is none.

A submersible pressure gauge functions like a gas gauge in a car. If the diver fails to check the gauge periodically during the dive, an out of air situation can occur without the diver realizing it until it is too late. On a deep dive, this can have disastrous consequences.

Depth Gauges

Depth gauges are instruments designed to be used in conjunction with a diver's watch to calculate the diver's maximum allowable bottom time. In the 1960s and early 70s almost every diver used a depth gauge, but today, the depth gauge has been largely replaced by the dive computer.

Some depth gauges have a maximum depth indicating needle that can be reset by the diver at the start of each dive. If the general depth range of the diver at the time of a diving accident is known, and the depth gauge is equipped with this feature, it will sometimes suggest the depth at which the accident took place. However, depending on the circumstances of the accident, the information supplied by this device will not always be reliable. For example, unless you know the needle was reset prior to the dive when the accident occurred, the reading may come from a prior dive.

Almost all older depth gauges were mechanical devices that were prone to failure if not properly maintained.

Dive Computers

To help avoid decompression sickness, sport divers traditionally relied upon decompression calculations pro-

vided in the form of printed "tables" to compute their allowable bottom time for a particular depth and series of dives. These calculations were not difficult to perform, but unless done frequently, the process was error prone. Even divers well versed in the use of the tables made mistakes in their calculations.

In the early 1980s, the microprocessor had developed to the point where it was possible to design a device that could be programmed to take the data input from a pressure transducer and calculate decompression schedules based upon depth readings and the time spent at these depths. The modern dive computer was first developed during this period as a device that could be worn by the diver to automatically calculate the diver's decompression status.

Dive computers are the modern equivalent of the aircraft's black box. Today's dive computers can be as small as a wrist watch and contain many powerful functions.

Most dive computers make their calculations based upon a mathematical formula known as an "algorithm." Different manufacturers use different algorithms

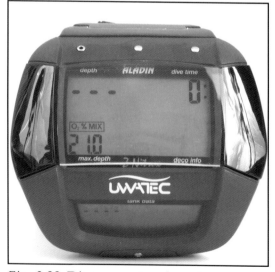

Fig. 3.22 Dive computers have become very sophisticated. This model receives tank pressure via a wireless transmitter connected to the regulator.

so comparisons of dive profiles from one computer to another cannot be made.

The calculations made by dive computers cannot be relied upon in all cases to help a diver avoid decompression sickness. The computer does not make calculations based upon what physiological events are taking place in the diver's body. Even if the diver follows the calculations made by the computer precisely, there is the possibility that decompression sickness will still occur. There are too many biologic variations in each dive for a dive computer to provide decompression calculations that are 100% safe. Some of the variables that have been suggested to be associated with DCS are:

- Water temperature
- Work load during the dive
- Adequacy of the thermal protection worn by the diver
- The amount of body fat the diver carries
- Use of alcohol prior to the dive
- The diver's age

However, it is important to note that none of these factors has been clearly shown to affect the incidence of DCS on a given dive.

Some dive computers are very "aggressive" in the amount of bottom time they allow the diver, and the short length of the surface intervals they require between dives. Other computers are much more conservative. In a decompression incident, it may be important to determine what algorithm was used and what impact this may have had on the diver's sequence of dives.

There have been lawsuits that involve divers who suffer from decompression sickness while using a dive computer at the time of their injury. In some cases, the diver failed to understand the proper techniques for using the computer, or failed to follow proper procedures for using the computer even though he under-

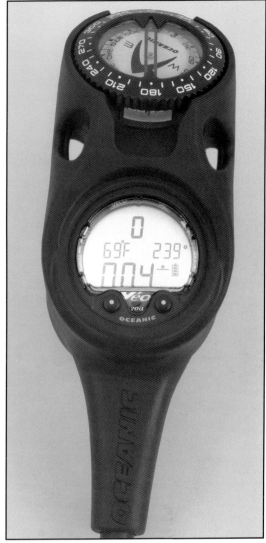

Fig. 3.23 This dive computer is "air integrated" and includes an electronic air pressure gauge.

stood the computer's limitations. In other cases, the diver followed the computer's recommendations precisely, but still suffered from decompression sickness. In still other cases, there were computer failures or errors programming the underlying algorithm. It is always possible for a dive computer to fail through improper battery replacement.

Depending on the make and model, a dive computer may be capable of supplying some, or all, of the following information:

- Time of the dive, including descent,

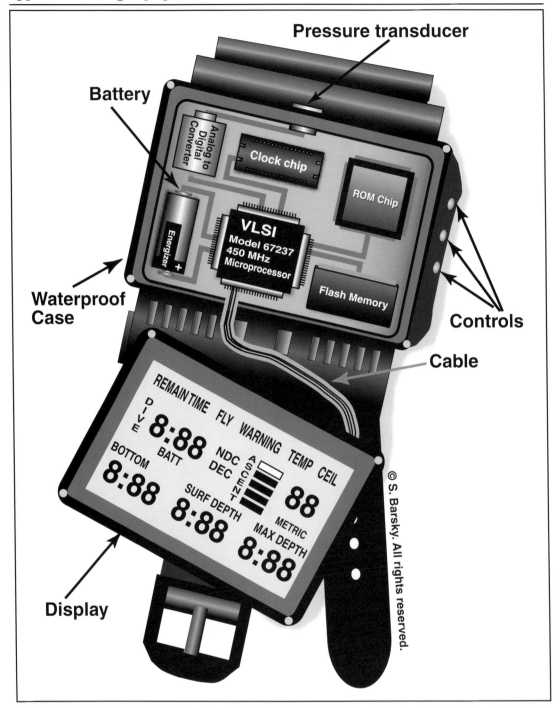

Pressure transducer

Battery

Analog to Digital Converter

Clock chip

ROM Chip

VLSI
Model 67237
450 MHz
Microprocessor

Energizer +

Flash Memory

Waterproof Case

Controls

Cable

REMAIN TIME FLY WARNING TEMP CEIL
DIVE
8:88
BATT
NDC
DEC
ASCENT
BOTTOM
8:88
SURF DEPTH
8:88
88
METRIC
MAX DEPTH
8:88

Display

© S. Barsky. All rights reserved.

Fig. 3.24 Cutaway drawing of a "typical" dive computer. There are numerous different designs on the market today.

bottom time, and ascent
- Maximum depth
- Average depth
- Depth during any given point during the dive
- Air consumption rate including starting and ending air pressure

in the diver's cylinder
- Water temperature during the dive
- Rapid ascent indication
- Decompression information

Many modern dive computers are designed to interface with a personal computer so that the information from the dive can be downloaded. This information can be critical in evaluating what took place during a dive. The information can usually be printed out in a graphical format that is easy to interpret.

Rebreathers

A rebreather is a type of diving gear that is designed to recirculate each breath the diver takes, remove the exhaled carbon dioxide gas, and replenish the oxygen. This type of diving equipment is generally more complex, expensive, and maintenance intensive than open-circuit diving gear.

Rebreathers also require specialized training. Unlike open-circuit equipment, the training for each different type of rebreather is unique and specific to that unit. Even experienced diving accident investigators would undoubtedly find it difficult to spot a problem with a specific model of rebreather unless they had been trained in the use of that exact model. Military, scientific, technical, and some sport divers commonly use rebreathers.

The type of rebreather primarily used by sport divers is the semi-closed circuit rebreather, which is the simplest equip-

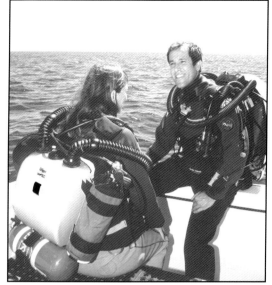

Fig. 3.25 Rebreathers require specialized training beyond what is available in an ordinary scuba course.

ment of this type. They have no electronic controls and are relatively inexpensive. They are usually designed to utilize "nitrox," a gas mixture containing nitrogen and oxygen in a ratio that contains more oxygen than normal air. The semi-closed circuit rebreather is the most commonly encountered type of rebreather in sport diving. These systems are generally

Risk Recognition for Divers and Diving Professionals

In the setting of an accident, the three items of recreational diving equipment that are of most concern are buoyancy compensators (especially the power inflator mechanism), dive computers, and dry suits. In the event of an accident involving these pieces of equipment, it is imperative that the diver, the dive store, and the manufacturer followed the appropriate industry standards for training and use of the product.

Not all buoyancy compensators use the same diameter hoses. Care should be taken not to install an inflator mechanism that is too large for a smaller diameter hose.

It is extremely important that diving retailers be careful in regards to how they sell or promote these items. For example, many dive stores have sold dive computers to professional seafood divers and touted them as the ultimate answer to their decompression problems. In fact, most dive computer manuals are careful to state that these devices are <u>not</u> intended for use by commercial divers.

Similarly, dive stores have sold dry suits without providing adequate instruction in the use of this type of equipment, and there have been accidents as a result. Although dry suits are relatively simple to use, divers who wear them need training to use them with a reasonable degree of safety.

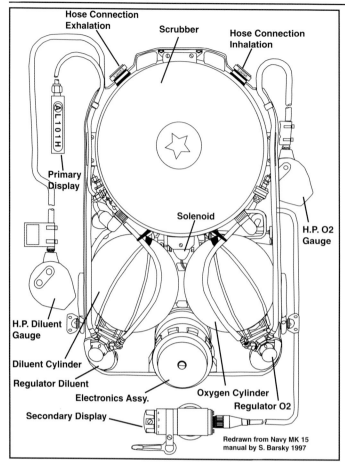

Hose Connection Exhalation
Scrubber
Hose Connection Inhalation
Primary Display
Solenoid
H.P. O2 Gauge
H.P. Diluent Gauge
Diluent Cylinder
Regulator Diluent
Electronics Assy.
Oxygen Cylinder
Regulator O2
Secondary Display
Redrawn from Navy MK 15 manual by S. Barsky 1997

Fig. 3.26 Rebreathers are much more complicated than ordinary open-circuit scuba. Each diver must know how to maintain his own unit.

not used at depths below 130 feet of sea water (FSW). However, end users can and do use gas mixtures that were not designed to be used with these systems to extend their range to greater depths.

Fully closed-circuit rebreathers can be designed to use either pure oxygen or other gas mixtures. Rebreathers designed to use pure oxygen are typically used by the military or scientific divers in limited applications. A few sport divers use this type of rebreather, but the depth limitation for this type of gear is only 25 feet due to the dangers involved in breathing pure oxygen at deeper depths.

Fully closed-circuit electronic rebreathers have military, scientific, and sport diving applications. These are the most sophisticated type of rebreathers. They have been used to depths in excess of 400 FSW. At depths below 200 FSW, these systems automatically mix helium and oxygen to provide the proper combi-nations of breathing gas.

One of the most important safety features of all rebreathers (with the exception of the pure oxygen models) is an oxygen monitoring system. If the rebreather is supplying too little oxygen, the diver may suffer from "hypoxia" and pass out. If the rebreather is supplying too much oxygen at depth, the diver can develop oxygen poisoning and go into convulsions. Either situation can lead to drowning.

There have been a number of rebreather accidents in the sport diving community. Most of these accidents were due to poor maintenance or improper use of the rebreather.

Alternate Air Sources

Scuba divers normally carry some type of emergency breathing system in order to share air with another diver, or to provide themselves with their own in-dependent back-up air supply.

In its simplest form, an "octopus rig" is simply an extra hose and mouthpiece connected to a diver's own regulator. This device is used to provide emergency air to another scuba diver whose own air supply has been exhausted. There is some skill required to use these systems and accidents have occurred, particularly when the diver who is providing the air to the diver in distress has run out of air, too.

To provide personal security in the event of an emergency at depth, some divers elect to carry a small, completely redundant scuba system. "Spare-Air®" is a compact, commercial product with a tiny cylinder of air and a regulator that is permanently attached to the cylinder. Both high and low-pressure stages of the regulator are contained in a single unit. A diver can use Spare-Air® as their own emergency supply, or can hand it off to another diver without being physically attached to them in any way.

Wreck and cave divers may carry completely redundant, small scuba cylinders known as "pony bottles" with fully equipped regulator systems. They may also carry additional full–size cylinders that are hung from their diving harness and are referred to as "sling bottles." These bottles are generally used during the decompression phase of a technical dive and frequently contain a high per-

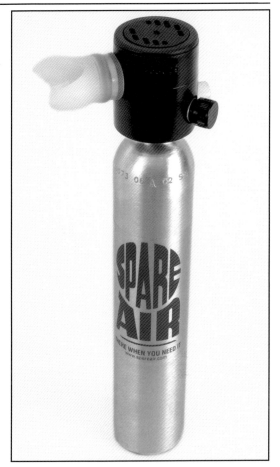

Fig. 3.28 Spare Air® is a completely self-contained independent air source used by some divers in out-of-air emergencies.

centage of oxygen to hasten decompression. A number of fatalities have occurred when technical divers have used the wrong gas mixture (usually containing too much oxygen) at deeper depths.

Full-Face Masks

Full-face masks combine a sport diving mask that covers the eyes and nose, with the regulator that supplies the breathing gas, into a single, integrated system. No part of the diver's face is exposed to the water. With either a full-face mask or a helmet, the diver does not need to hold the mouthpiece in his mouth. There is a space in the mask known as an "oral-nasal cavity" that covers the nose and mouth. The oral-nasal cavity helps to reduce any build-up of carbon dioxide

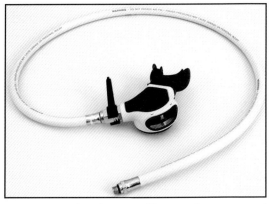

Fig. 3.27 This low profile regulator second stage is designed to be used as an "octopus" to supply breathing gas for an out-of-air dive partner.

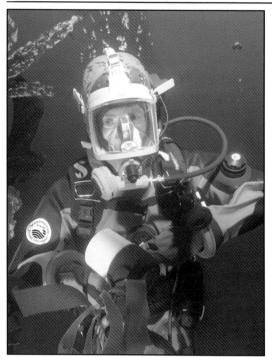

Fig. 3.29 Full-face masks cover the eyes, nose, and mouth of the diver. They incorporate the regulator and provide a way to talk.

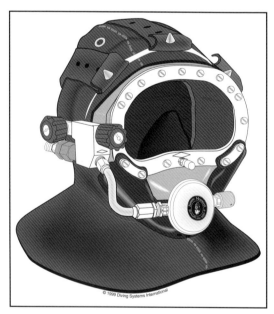

Fig. 3.30 Commercial divers use heavy-duy full-face masks like this one which has a fiberglass frame and a Lexan® face port. (© Kirby Morgan Dive Systems, Inc. All rights reserved.)

in the mask (i.e., decreases "dead-air" space) and provides a place to mount the microphone that is used for communications.

The essential components of a full-face mask include a frame for mounting the hardware and lens, a rubber face seal that connects to the frame to keep the water out of the mask, and a regulator to adjust the air pressure to that equal to the depth of the diver. There may also be additional devices built into (or attached) to the mask to assist the diver in equalizing his ears, provide communications, and connect emergency breathing systems known as "bail-out" systems.

Some full-face masks are lightweight systems designed primarily for sport diving. Masks for this purpose are not as robustly built or as heavy as masks that are built for commercial diving applications. Some of the masks used for sport diving include those made by Kirby Morgan Dive Systems and Neptune Systems. The Interspiro Divator Mark II and the EXO-26® are masks that are used primarily by public safety divers, but are also used by some sport divers.

One of the most heavy-duty full-face mask is the Kirby-Morgan Band Mask® which is used primarily for commercial diving. The frame for the mask is fiberglass, the lens is made of Lexan®, and the hardware is all stainless steel or chrome plated brass. An attached hood provides warmth and has pockets for mounting the earphones that are used for communications. The hood is made from wetsuit material and is not designed to keep the diver's head dry.

One of the major advantages of a full-face mask or helmet is that a diver who has lost consciousness underwater will probably not inhale water if he is wearing this equipment. On the negative side, with most masks of this type, unless it is rigged to accept a secondary breathing gas source, in most cases the diver will need to remove the mask in order to breathe from another air source. Once the diver removes the mask, he is effectively "blind" underwater, an undesirable situation at any time, but particularly so during an emergency.

Wireless Communications

While a full-mask facilitates speech underwater by eliminating the mouthpiece and providing an air cavity into which the diver may talk, the mask itself has no apparatus to amplify or transmit speech through the water. For two scuba divers to be able to communicate with each other, both must be equipped with some type of electronic underwater communications system. Since it is impractical and unsafe for two free-swimming divers to be connected together by a wire, these systems are designed to provide "wireless communications."

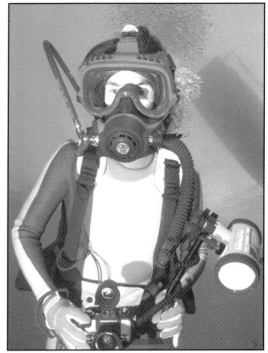

Fig. 3.31 Full-face masks are widely used by diving scientists, public safety divers, and commercial divers. Some sport divers use them, too.

Wireless communications will allow divers to communicate at distances up to about 1500 feet. However, there are many factors that may interfere with the effectiveness of a wireless system including wrecks, seaweed, differences in water temperature, and even the type of suit the diver is wearing.

Although today's wireless communications systems are very effective, they are not as reliable as hard-wired systems, where there is a wire connecting the diver's mask to a special communications box on the surface. However, in many situations, a hard-wired system is not practical and wireless communications must be used.

Diving Helmets

Diving helmets are used by professional divers and commercial divers and rarely, if ever, by recreational divers. Their weight, expense, and complexity are far beyond what is practical for sport diving.

Helmets differ from full-face masks in that a helmet is designed to enclose

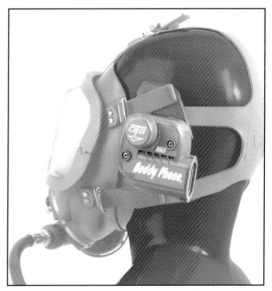

Fig. 3.32 The ability to use wireless communications, like the system mounted on the side of this mask, is one of the main reasons to use a full-face mask. (© Ocean Technology Systems, Inc. All rights reserved.)

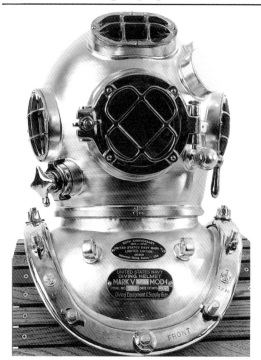

Fig. 3.33 It's rare to see traditional heavy-gear helmets in use anymore.

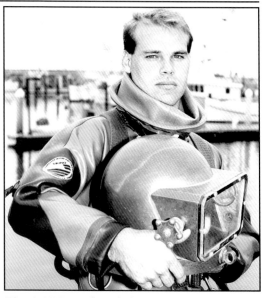

Fig. 3.35 Free-flow helmets are much simpler in design that demand helmets. A low-pressure compressor is required to supply the air for this type of helmet.

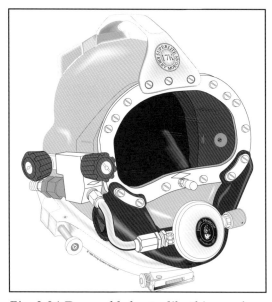

Fig. 3.34 Demand helmets, like this one, have a regulator built into them. (© Kirby Morgan Dive Systems, Inc. All rights reserved.)

the diver's entire head and keep it dry as well. The helmet also provides mechanical protection from falling objects or physical impact. Since the communications components are kept dry and the helmet is sealed around the diver's neck

rather than the face, speech intelligibility is greatly improved. In commercial diving, helmets are frequently equipped with lights and small television cameras that can relay a picture to the topside support team.

There are two main categories of diving helmets. "Free-flow helmets" have no regulator mounted on the helmet. The air is supplied in a continuous flow of breathing gas into the helmet, so that the pressure inside the helmet is always slightly higher than the surrounding water pressure. This type of helmet requires a low-pressure compressor to supply the volume of gas required to use it safely.

"Demand helmets" have a second stage regulator built into them. Like a scuba regulator, these helmets only supply breathing gas when the diver demands it, i.e., inhales through the regulator, although they are equipped with valves that can be turned on or off to provide a steady flow of gas to defog the lens or clear the helmet of water in the event that it floods.

Diving helmets consist of two main components, i.e., the yoke/neck dam that seals around the diver's neck and clamps to the bottom of the helmet, and the helmet itself. Most helmets can be connected to dry suits via the yoke to help protect the diver in polluted water.

All diving helmets and full-face masks used for surface-supplied diving must be equipped with a "non-return" valve to prevent air from rushing back up the hose to a lower pressure in the event the hose is severed. If this valve is missing or should it not work, the diver may be subject to a "squeeze," which is the result of a difference in pressure between the inside of the helmet and the environment.

Diving helmet failures are usually due to poor maintenance. The helmets themselves are extremely rugged, but are generally subject to abuse in the commercial diving environment. End user modifications to helmets and their yokes have resulted in fatalities.

In the past decade, "counterfeit" helmets have been manufactured in China that do not have the same quality or meet the original specifications of the true product. In the investigation of an accident, the uninitiated may have a difficult time separating a counterfeit helmet from the real product.

Bail-Out Systems

Divers who use surface-supplied air diving systems also will frequently use a "bail-out system," which is a diver-worn emergency breathing gas system that connects directly to the full-face mask or helmet. The bail-out system allows the diver to switch to this emergency supply should the air supply from the surface be lost. This system is similar to the pony bottle used by sport divers. Bail-out bottles are required under industry standards (ADCI Consensus Standards) except in situations where space does not permit them to be worn.

Bail-out systems consist of a small (or large) scuba cylinder with a first stage regulator, connected to the diving helmet via a short hose or "whip." The first stage regulator should be fitted with an over-pressure relief valve so that in the event the regulator begins to "creep" or build pressure above its normal setting, the hose will not burst.

Support Equipment
High-pressure Air Compressors

Although few scuba divers own personal high-pressure air compressors,

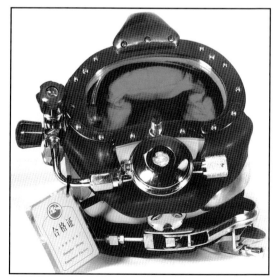

Fig. 3.36 Is it real or is it fake? This is an unlicensed Chinese counterfeit of the popular SuperLite-17® diving helmet.

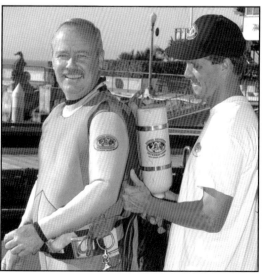

Fig. 3.37 Divers who use surface-supplied gear are wise to wear a bail-out bottle whenever possible.

all dive stores, diving resorts, and large dive boats will generally have at least one high-pressure compressor and sometimes more than one for filling scuba cylinders. These compressors may be powered by gasoline or diesel engines, or by electrical motors.

By the nature of their operation, compressors are subject to high heat, vibration, and pressure changes within the cylinders, piping, and hoses. High-pressure compressors deliver air at pressures that may reach as high as 3000 pounds per square inch (p.s.i.) or more. Components of compressors can fail causing injuries to anyone who is nearby as parts fly about.

Due to the increased use of special gas mixtures known as nitrox (containing higher than normal percentages of oxygen) in recreational diving, fires and explosions can occur at dive stores that pump these mixtures. High-pressure oxygen and petroleum products are a volatile combination. There have been explosions and fires in dive stores as a result of the improper handling of high-pressure oxygen.

High-pressure compressor operators maintain a log of compressor hours, oil and filter changes, and breathing air filter changes. In addition, the air should be sampled and tested for purity by a reputable testing laboratory on a regular basis. The testing laboratory will provide

the user with a certificate confirming the quality of the air.

The air pumped by a high-pressure air compressor can be the direct cause of a diving accident in several ways. If the operator allows the intake of the compressor to draw in carbon monoxide gas, (which is created by gasoline and diesel engines) the diver can be subjected to carbon monoxide poisoning, which can be fatal.

Oil lubricated compressors that are inadequately maintained or running poorly may allow small amounts of oil to leak past the rings of the compressor. These small amounts of oil, when subjected to the heat and pressure of the compressor's cylinder, may produce carbon monoxide.

Another less common type of "accident" occurs when an oil lubricated compressor is improperly maintained and large amounts of oil leak past the rings of the compressor and are vaporized in the compressed air. Divers who inhale this oily air may suffer from a condition known as "lipoid pneumonia."

Low-pressure Air Compressors

Low-pressure air compressors are used by the commercial diving industry to provide compressed air for surface-supplied air diving and for the operation of decompression chambers. These compressors can also pump carbon monoxide to the diver if they aren't correctly set up.

Low-pressure compressors are typically used with a "volume tank" that acts as a reservoir or "reserve" of air for the surface-supplied diver. The volume tank also acts as a "water trap" to collect the moisture in the breathing air, and will have a valve fitted to the lowest part of the cylinder to drain off this excess water. The volume tank/compressor system will usually have some type of filter to help remove contaminants from the breathing air. Volume tanks must be ASME (American Society of Mechanical Engineers) approved. They should also be equipped with a check valve on the

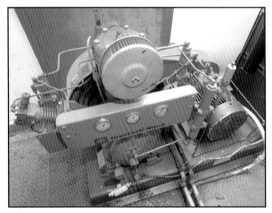

Fig. 3.38 High-pressure compressors for breathing air require special filtration and the air they pump should be analyzed regularly.

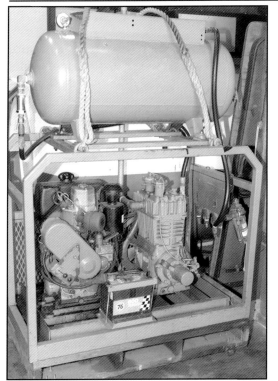

Fig. 3.39 Low-pressure compressors are used for surface-supplied diving and to operate hyperbaric chambers.

Most communications boxes are powered by batteries and have no provision for connecting 110-volt power. It's possible with a system that is improperly wired or grounded to send shipboard power down through the communication wire to the diver.

When a diver is breathing a gas mixture containing helium and oxygen (heliox) at depth, his speech will be seriously distorted and may sound somewhat like Donald Duck. "Helium unscramblers" are special communications boxes designed to modify the sound of a diver's speech when they are breathing helium-oxygen gas mixtures at depth to make it sound more normal. Without an unscrambler, it can be difficult to understand some divers. Experienced diving supervisors often turn off the unscrambling feature of these boxes so that they will be better able to understand the diver in the event the unscrambler fails.

inlet side, a pressure gauge, and a relief valve.

Just as the air from a high-pressure compressor must be sampled on a regular basis, the air from a low-pressure compressor must be checked as well.

Communications Boxes

For divers using full-face masks or diving helmets with breathing gas supplied by a hose from the surface, a communications box is an essential piece of equipment for the diver to speak with his topside support team. The box acts as an amplifier to the signal that is carried by the communications wire attached to the hose and will include a speaker and volume controls. Some boxes will support multiple divers and provide what is known as a "cross-talk" capability. There are also special boxes that allow a topside divemaster to communicate with free-swimming divers using wireless communications.

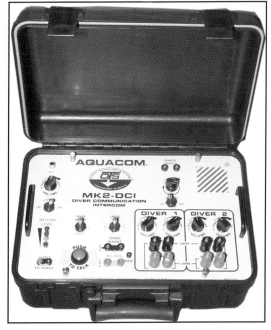

Fig. 3.40 Hard-wire communications are the preferred method for the surface-support crew to communicate with a commercial diver working underwater.

Breathing Gas Manifolds

There are more components to a surface-supplied air diving system than there are to a hookah system, even though they work in a very similar way. In a surface-supplied air diving system, there is a control manifold that is used to monitor the diver's air supply and depth. The manifold also allows more than one air supply to be hooked up at a time, so that the topside personnel can switch to a different air supply should the primary supply fail for any reason, or should a different gas mixture be needed for decompression.

For diving with mixtures of helium and oxygen, a special "mixed-gas diving manifold" is normally used. The manifold is typically designed to accept mixed gas from at least two, and as many as three, independent banks of gas cylinders. The high-pressure gas enters the manifold and the pressure is reduced through a regulator. Most manifolds have redundant regulators so that if one fails,

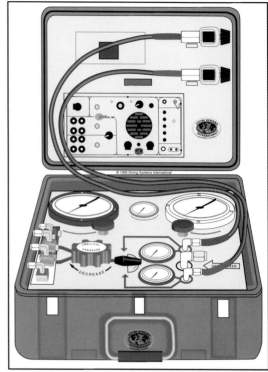

Fig. 3.41 *This portable air diving manifold contains everything needed to run the dive in a single box. (© Kirby Morgan Dive Systems, Inc. All rights reserved.)*

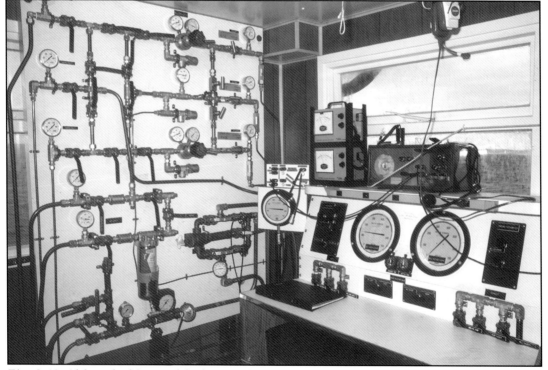

Fig. 3.42 *Although this panel looks complex, it's relatively simple to operate. The plumbing shown here is capable of running air, mixed gas, and bell/saturation dives. It also includes a hot-water mixing system for the diver's suit.*

another may be immediately put on line. In addition, the mixed gas manifold will also accept air, usually from a low-pressure source. Modified mixed-gas manifolds can also be used to run dives made from diving bells.

Most breathing gas manifolds include a system known as a "pneumofathometer system" for checking the diver's depth from topside. The system includes a needle valve, a highly accurate gauge, and a fitting to connect to a small diameter air hose. Air enters the system through the needle valve, flows through the gauge, and then is routed down the hose to the diver. When the air exits the open end of the "pneumo hose," the diver notifies topside that air is flowing or that he "has bubbles." The operator topside closes the needle valve at the manifold and the air pressure that is trapped in the hose provides a reading on the gauge of the diver's depth.

Breathing gas manifolds are extremely reliable and it is rare for one to fail. More often, they can be a contributing factor in an accident when mistakes are made in their use.

The breathing gas manifold may also be referred to as "the rack," and the person who operates it, if they are not the diving supervisor, will usually be referred to as the "rack operator."

Umbilicals

The basic diver's umbilical consists of a minimum of three members; i.e., a breathing gas hose to supply air or mixed-gas to the diver, a pneumo hose, and a communications wire. The hoses may be "married" with tape, wrapped with plastic shrink tubing, or specially twisted, to keep the various lines together.

Additional hoses and cables that may be added or included in the umbilical include:

- Strength member – designed to give added strength to the bundle.
- Hot water hose – an insulated hose

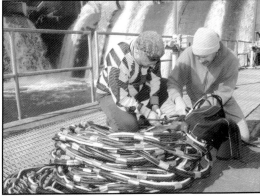

Fig. 3.43 Divers' umbilicals are heavy and bulky.

that supplies hot water to the diver for his suit
- Television wire – for relaying a video image from the diver to topside
- Electrical power – 12 volt DC power travels down this cable to provide power to a light mounted on the diver's mask or helmet

Diving hoses may be designed to either float or sink. Public safety divers and seafood divers tend to use floating hoses because they are easier to manage and less prone to becoming "fouled" (snagged) on the bottom. Conversely, commercial divers tend to use sinking hoses, which are generally more rugged.

Umbilicals themselves rarely cause trouble, although fittings can fail if abused, as can the hose itself. A more common type of accident occurs when a diver is using a floating hose and a passing vessel snags the hose, dragging the diver to the surface too quickly and causing decompression problems or direct trauma.

Diving Stage

On most small vessels, the easiest way for a diver to enter the water is to jump over the side of the boat. To board the vessel, a ladder is used in most cases.

For commercial diving operations on larger vessels, where there is a substantial distance to the water, it is usually im-

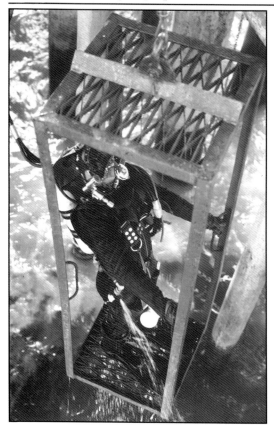

Fig. 3.44 Diving stages are used to hoist commercial divers out of the water in situations where a ladder is impractical or dangerous.

practical, and often unsafe, for the diver to use a ladder to climb back aboard. In these situations, most operations will use a diving "stage" to lower the diver to the water and hoist him back aboard.

Diving stages are usually made from either aluminum or steel, and are designed to support the diver and the weight of his equipment, in an open "cage." The stage will have a lifting eye on top of it for attaching a wire from a small crane or "davit" to lift the diver off the deck and lower him to the water or recover him. Lift wires for these davits may be improperly rigged or fail due to stress or corrosion.

In normal use, the stage is lowered over the side until it is just a few feet below the surface and the diver exits the stage to do his work. The stage is then normally recovered back aboard the deck of the boat so that it is available if the

need arises to put the stand-by diver in the water. If visibility is poor, or there are strong currents, the diver's hose may be deliberately fed through the stage prior to the start of the dive, so that his support crew can pull the diver back to the stage.

Most stages are overbuilt and rarely if ever fail. A more likely type of accident occurs when a diver enters a stage to return to the ship, but fails to ensure that his hose is clear of any obstructions in the water. In this type of situation, the diver may be pulled out of the stage by his own hose.

Open Bottom Bell

An open bottom bell is a diving stage with a cover over the top quarter or third of the unit. The purpose of the cover is to provide an air pocket in an emergency in case the diver's mask or helmet fails during a deep dive that requires decompression. At least one emergency breathing gas cylinder with a regulator attached to it is mounted on the outside of this type of stage.

When divers are doing deep, surface-supplied dives, i.e., using mixed-gas in excess of 165 FSW, the stage is usually lowered to the diver's depth, so that the diver has the security of the covered "bell" in the event of an emergency. This is a fairly standard procedure.

Decompression Chambers

A decompression chamber is a pressure vessel that is designed to safely hold humans under pressure for the purposes of performing decompression following a dive, treating decompression sickness, and conducting hyperbaric oxygen therapy. These devices are classified under a code by the American Society of Mechanical Engineers (ASME) known as "PVHO," or Pressure Vessel for Human Occupancy.

There are many terms that are used to refer to decompression chambers, including recompression chambers, hyperbaric

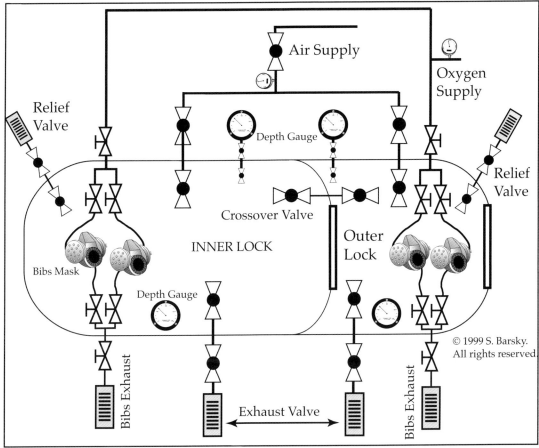

Fig. 3.45 In commercial diving, the philosophy for plumbing most decompression chambers is that each external valve should be matched by a similar control on the inside of the chamber. This schematic shows the arrangement of a "typical" decompression chamber.

chambers, and just plain "chambers." Although you may hear people argue about which term is correct, any of these terms is acceptable.

In the commercial diving field, almost all decompression chambers are made from steel and designed to be "portable," meaning they can be lifted with a crane and moved with a flat bed truck. To operate the chamber to treat a diver, additional equipment is needed including a low-pressure compressor, a communications box, and a supply of high-pressure oxygen.

Chambers are plumbed with a variety of fittings that are made primarily from copper, brass, and stainless steel. The purpose of the valves on the chamber is to either feed air, or oxygen, into the chamber and to let air, or oxygen, out of the chamber. On a chamber designed for use by commercial divers, in most cases, every valve that is on the outside of the chamber is duplicated on the inside of the chamber. The rationale for this is so that the diver inside can run his own decompression in an emergency.

Chambers are also normally fitted with special "thru-hull" penetrators to carry communications wire, and sometimes electrical power for lighting, into the chamber. Although it is rare, if these penetrators fail, the chamber can depressurize.

Most chambers are fitted with two compartments or "locks" and two doors or "hatches." These doors are usually referred to as the inner hatch and the outer hatch. Dual compartment chambers are commonly known as "double lock chambers." The "inner" lock is where the diver is treated or decompressed, while the outer lock is used to transfer personnel and equipment in and out of the chamber.

The most serious type of chamber accident that can occur is a chamber fire, where oxygen in the chamber supports rapid combustion. Although this type of incident is rare, it is extremely serious when it occurs. Most chambers are fitted with oxygen analyzers to monitor the level of oxygen in the chamber to ensure it does not get too high. In addition, most chambers are fitted with special masks, known as "BIBS" for the divers to wear while breathing oxygen. These masks are designed to "dump" oxygen "overboard," i.e., out of the chamber rather than exhaust into the chamber itself. BIBS is an acronym which stands for "Built-In Breathing System."

One chamber fire that occurred in California took place when a commercial diver entered a chamber, that had not been properly vented, and lit a cigarette. The oxygen in the chamber supported combustion of all of the flammable items inside the chamber, including the diver's clothes, hair, eyebrows, and ears. Although the diver survived the fire, today his ears are little more than stubs on the side of his head.

Diving Bells

A closed diving bell is a steel cylinder that is fitted with special valves and other fittings to provide a safe, dry haven for a diver under pressure. Like decompression chambers, diving bells are fitted with hatches on the inside and the outside, but the outer hatch of the bell seals with external pressure, while the inner hatch of the bell seals with internal pressure. Between the two hatches is a short "trunk" which also must be equalized to permit the transfer of divers under pressure from the bell into a decompression chamber. Diving bells are also considered Pressure Vessels for Human Occupancy (PVHO).

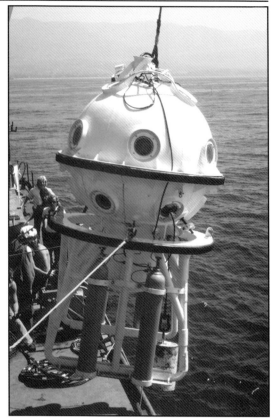

Fig. 3.46 Diving bells are manufactured in a variety of shapes and sizes, but the two most common are the spherical bell shown here and cylindrical shape shown on the facing page.

Most bells are so small that there is barely room for two divers, their umbilicals and helmets. Any special tools that the diver may need are either hung on the outside of the bell, or lowered to the diver on a line, once the bell reaches the bottom depth.

The bell has its own special umbilical, which provides it with breathing gas, electrical power, and hot water for heating. Manifolds outside and inside the bell route the breathing gas and hot water to shorter, smaller diameter umbilicals that are used to supply the divers. Most bells are also equipped with an emergency power system and some quantity of emergency breathing gas. A "drop weight system" with ditchable weights provides the ballast required for the bell to submerge. An emergency transponder must be mounted on the outside of the bell so

Mask drawings © Kirby Morgan Dive Systems, Inc. All rights reserved.

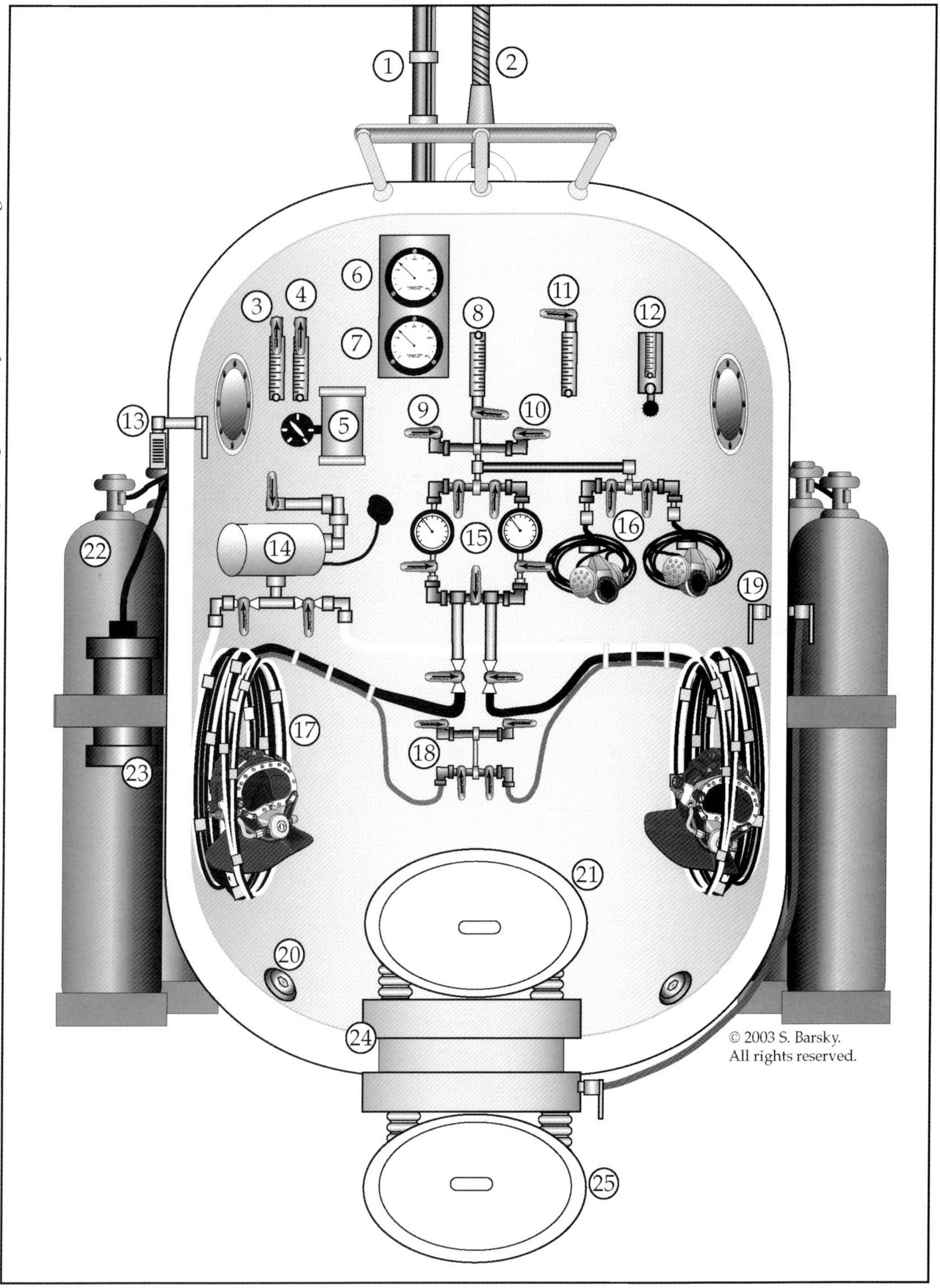

© 2003 S. Barsky.
All rights reserved.

Fig. 3.47 Components of a "typical" diving bell: 1) Umbilical 2) main lift wire 3) topside controlled exhaust 4) topside controlled (gas) supply 5) carbon dioxide scrubber 6) external depth gauge 7) internal depth gauge 8) bell blow down 9) main gas supply control 10) emergency gas supply 11) bell controlled exhaust 12) oxygen make-up flowmeter 13) relief valve   14) bell heater 15) divers supply manifold 16) BIBs manifold 17) diver's umbilical and mask 18) pneumo supply 19) trunk equalization 20) drop weight control mechanism 21) upper hatch 22) emergency gas bottle 23) emergency power supply 24) trunk (manway) 25) bottom hatch.

Types of Diving Equipment

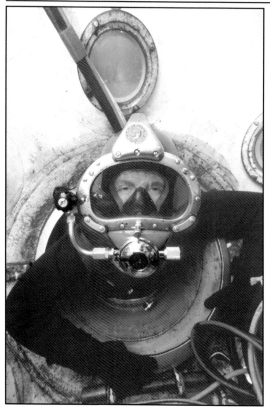

Fig. 3.48 On a normal job, a saturation diver will usually work a four hour shift in the water before returning to the diving bell.

that it can be located in an emergency, should it be separated from its lift wire and umbilical.

A special "bell handling system" is needed to put the bell into the water and recover it. The most common designs are simple davits and "u-booms." Some type of winch is always part of the system.

Since the outer hatch seals with external pressure, a diving bell can be lowered to depth while its interior remains at surface pressure. This procedure is used on many dives, where the bell, with the divers inside, is lowered to depth unpressurized, and then "blown down" to bottom pressure once the divers are at the job site.

The normal operating procedure for any bell dive is to have one diver inside the bell tending the hose for the diver working in the water. The tender inside the bell also serves as the standby diver to go to the aid of the diver in the water

in the event of an emergency. Topside can communicate with both the diver in the bell and the diver in the water. However, in some bells, the tender in the bell cannot hear the diver in the water. Most bells have viewports so the tender in the bell can see the diver outside.

At the completion of the first diver's work period, which may last four hours or more, he returns to the bell to switch places with the second diver, who also completes a four-hour stint outside. Once the second diver has completed his work, he returns to the bell. Both hatches are closed and the bell is brought directly to the surface. By closing the inner hatch and raising the bell quickly, the inner hatch seals the bell and maintains the inside pressure, while the bell ascends to a shallower depth. Meanwhile the pressure inside the bell is reduced at a slow rate, according to the divers' decompression schedule, which may take many hours or days. Once the bell is back on the deck of the ship, it can be connected to a decompression chamber that has a mating connection for the trunk of the bell. The divers can then transfer into the decompression chamber where they can complete the remainder of their decompression in relative comfort and safety.

Diving bells can be used at any depth, but generally they are not used until the water depth exceeds 165 FSW. The decision to use a bell takes into account many factors, but primarily will be determined by the depth and bottom time needed to complete the work.

There are many different types of accidents that may occur involving diving bells. One of the most serious accidents that can occur with a bell is a rapid loss of pressure or "explosive decompression." This has occurred when the connection between the bell and the decompression chamber on the deck of the ship has failed, either due to an accident such as an improperly tightened connection or a construction defect. This type of accident can have fatal consequences for the divers, who inevitably will suffer explosive decompression sickness, and the topside personnel, who may be struck by bolts or other objects.

Another serious bell diving accident occurs when the bell umbilical and lift wire for the bell are severed and the bell drops to the bottom. Unless the divers can ditch the drop weights, which isn't always possible, or the bell can be recovered in a reasonable period of time, the divers may die.

In the event of a rig fire or other disaster at sea, the bell may be the only means of evacuating the divers under pressure from a sinking ship. This is problematic, because unless the bell can be offloaded onto another vessel, it must be cast adrift, which usually will expose the divers to injury as the bell pitches about in heavy seas.

As with any piece of diving gear, improper maintenance can lead to an accident that can have fatal consequences.

Since the majority of the components of a diving system are custom made, maintaining these systems can be time consuming.

Saturation Systems

A saturation diving system is usually made up of either one very large decompression chamber, or a series of smaller chambers connected together, combined with a diving bell and other support equipment. The purpose of a saturation diving system is to support extended diving operations at deeper depths.

Aboard a saturation diving system, you will find almost every piece of diving gear listed here, with the exception of rebreathers and dive computers. Certain items may be greatly expanded, such as the breathing gas manifold, which may be part of a larger dive control van.

When divers live under pressure for extended periods they obviously require food and sanitation facilities. Accordingly, these chambers are fitted with

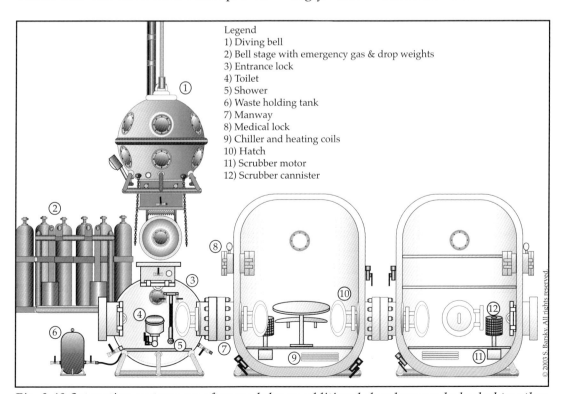

Legend
1) Diving bell
2) Bell stage with emergency gas & drop weights
3) Entrance lock
4) Toilet
5) Shower
6) Waste holding tank
7) Manway
8) Medical lock
9) Chiller and heating coils
10) Hatch
11) Scrubber motor
12) Scrubber cannister

© 2003 S. Barsky. All rights reserved.

Fig. 3.49 Saturation systems are often modular so additional chambers can be hooked together. The system shown here would only accommodate four divers, but could be enlarged.

special "medical locks," that are used to pass food and other necessities into and out of the chamber. In smaller chamber complexes, there may be no permanent toilet, and personal wastes may need to be locked out of the chamber in plastic bags. In larger complexes, there is usually a hard-plumbed toilet that may be flushed by filling the bowl with water and using chamber pressure to force the wastes through a valve out of the chamber.

Many years ago, a diver was nearly killed in an early saturation system through a mix-up in the use of the toilet and poor system design. In this case, the toilet seat did not have a gap so that when the diver sat on the toilet he made a seal on the rim with his body. Mistakenly, the toilet valve on the outside of the chamber was open when the diver opened the valve to flush the toilet, while he was still sitting on the bowl on the inside of the chamber. With the tremendous pressure differential from the interior of the chamber to the outside, the pressure forced the soft tissue of the diver's body into the toi-

let to fill the void, almost eviscerating the diver.

The diver managed to break the seal between the toilet seat and his body, gathered up his bleeding intestines which had exited his anus, and collapsed on the floor. A doctor was flown out from shore and operated on the diver in the chamber. The diver survived, but lost a large portion of his intestines and was forced to wear a colostomy bag from that time on.

Divers may live in a saturation system for periods of up to a month or more, making daily dives to complete large-scale projects. For example, saturation systems have been used to conduct complex salvage projects, the installation and removal of offshore oil platforms, repairs on dams, and other jobs of similar magnitude.

Life Support Modules (Environmental Control Unit)

A life support module, also known as an environmental control unit, is the system designed to maintain the proper tem-

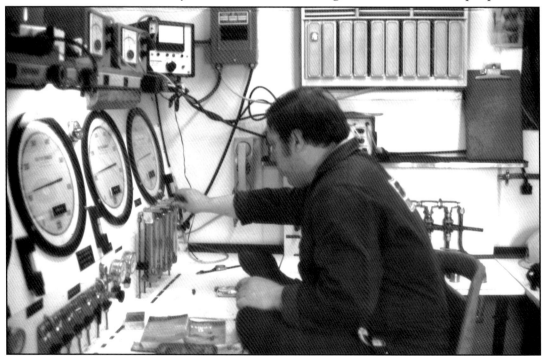

Fig. 3.50 It is the responsibility of the life support technician to monitor and adjust the oxygen levels, temperature and other parameters of the saturation system.

perature, humidity, oxygen, and carbon dioxide levels inside a saturation diving chamber complex. This system includes special heaters to warm the inside of the modules, and chillers that circulate cold water through coils in the bottom of the chamber to promote condensation and decrease the humidity of the environment.

On most saturation systems there will be a separate van devoted to the maintenance of the divers living in the chamber complex. A "life support technician" will be on duty 24 hours a day to care for the divers. It is the responsibility of the life support tech to monitor and adjust all of the following:

- Chamber depth and decompression
- Oxygen levels
- Carbon dioxide levels
- Temperature
- Humidity

In addition, the life support tech (or "sat tech") will also be responsible for seeing to it that the divers are fed and that sanitation needs are attended to, as well as maintaining a log of all events relating to the operation of the system.

Divers' Flags and Day Shapes

There are two types of divers' flags that are commonly used to alert other vessels that a diving operation is being conducted. They are the red and white sport diving flag and the blue and white Alpha flag used for commercial diving operations.

The red and white sport diving flag is commonly flown by sport diving charter boats and private vessels when sport divers are in the water. Although the red and white flag is well recognized by sport divers and many boat operators, as of 2003 it is not a legally recognized flag according to the *Navigation Rules International-Inland*, even though it has been in use for many years. Conversely, some states and local municipalities do recognize and re-

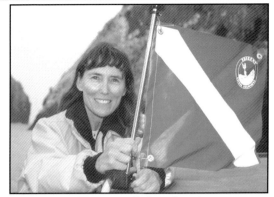

Fig. 3.51 The sport diving flag is not recognized in the Navigation Rules International-Inland.

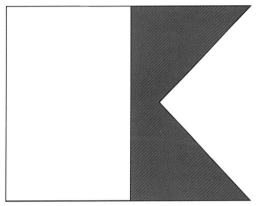

Fig. 3.52 The Alpha flag is required by the Navigation Rules International-Inland.

quire this flag.

The Alpha flag, which is blue and white in color, is required by the *Navigation Rules International-Inland*. This flag is used for commercial diving operations, and normally indicates submerged operations. Its meaning is, "I have a diver down; keep well clear and operate at slow speed." Some recreational dive boats fly both the Alpha flag and the sport diving flag.

Technically speaking, Rule 27 of the International Rules of the Road actually calls for a "rigid replica" of the Alpha flag, presumably so the "flag" can be seen when the wind is not blowing. In addition, whenever the size of a vessel engaged in diving makes it impracticable to exhibit all of the lights and shapes called for in section "D" of Rule 27, the rule calls for "three all-round lights in a vertical line where they can best be seen. The highest and lowest lights must be red and the middle light must be white. The rigid replica of the Alpha flag is used on a vessel where it is impractical to exhibit the day shapes that are normally used in submerged operations, also described in Rule 27.

The day shapes associated with submerged operations, but not necessarily diving are as follows:

• Two all-round red lights, or two balls, in a vertical line to indicate the side on which the obstruction exists;

• Two all-round green lights or two diamonds in a vertical line to indicate the side on which another vessel may pass;

• When at anchor the lights or shapes as described above are to be used.

The meaning of this combination of day shapes is ,"I am conducting a submerged operation. Keep well clear and operate at slow speed."

Any operation involving a commercial diver who is working using surface-supplied diving equipment must be identified as such through the use of the alpha flag and the appropriate day shapes. In a commercial operation involving the use of scuba, the sport diving flag is often flown as well.

Case History –Recreational Diving Accident

A sport diving charter boat was operating at night at an offshore island near the coast of California. The divers aboard were hunting for lobsters at night (lobsters come out of their holes at night and are much easier to catch).

One of the divers surfaced alone and reported that he had become separated from his dive partner. Roll call was taken and it was determined that the diver was in fact missing. There was no sign of the diver's lights that could be seen from the boat.

The vessel put out a mayday and alerted the U.S. Coast Guard as well as other vessels in the area. A search was made for the missing diver who was not located. After several hours, the dive boat pulled its anchor and headed for shore. Law enforcement authorities continued their search for the missing diver who still was not located the following day despite an intense search of the area.

Several weeks later, a recreational boat cruising along the coast saw a diver's body floating far offshore. They called the authorities who recovered the corpse.

An autopsy was conducted and the body was positively identified as the diver who had been previously missing. The autopsy concluded that the diver had suffered a bump on the head and that the cause of death was "drowning." The toxicology tests revealed that there was alcohol present in the blood.

The survivors of the diver filed a suit against the dive boat, contending that the boat had struck the diver, knocked him unconscious, and that he had drowned as a result. The defendants contended that there was no way to tell whether the diver was struck by the vessel or whether he had bumped his head on a rock or even another vessel. Whether the alcohol in the blood was caused by the diver consuming alcohol prior to his dive or due to decomposition was undetermined.

Ultimately, the case was settled outside of court.

Notes:

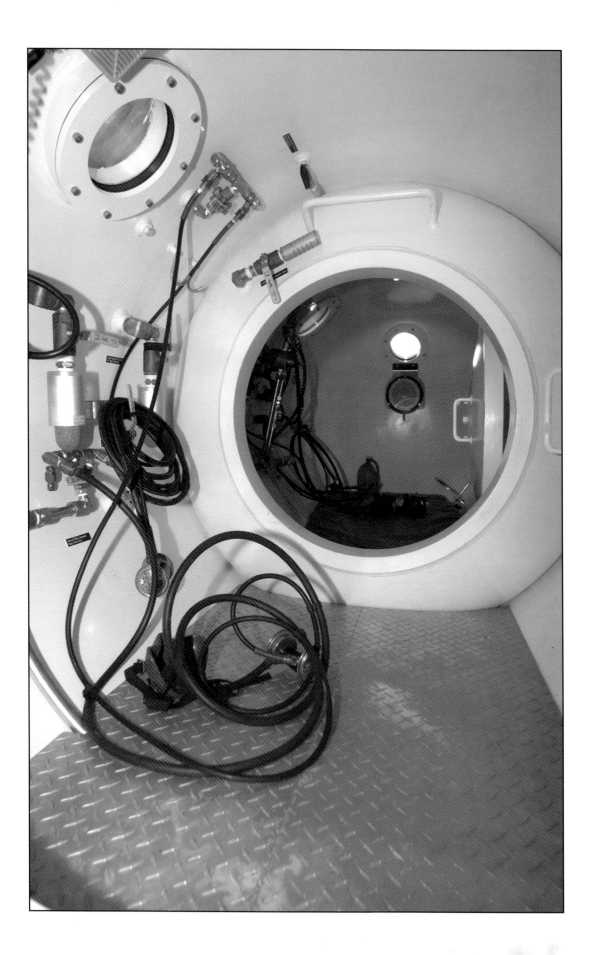

Chapter 4
Physiological Factors in Diving Accidents

There are numerous types of accidents that can cause death or serious injury to divers. They include drowning, lung over-pressure incidents, carbon monoxide poisoning, encounters with boats, and decompression sickness. In many cases, these factors may be combined, but the final cause of death will be attributed to a single cause. Other physiological factors may also cause diving accidents. These include hyperoxia (too high a level of oxygen), hypothermia and squeezes. These factors may all be primary causes of diving accidents.

Factors that may trigger a diving accident include hypothermia, nitrogen narcosis, dehydration, high breathing resistance, and exhaustion. With the exception of hypothermia, these factors will not usually be identified as a cause of death in a diving accident and may be completely overlooked as a contributing factor. Medical examiners and police investigators often do not have an understanding of diving and frequently do not get to see many diving accidents. As a result they will commonly reach the wrong conclusions in regards to the root cause of an accident.

Divers often die due to problems not directly related to diving, such as a cardiac event, which might be triggered due to a diver's poor physical condition and the high work loads that are sometimes associated with diving. All too often these deaths are ascribed to drowning.

Non-Fatal Diving Injuries
Squeezes

Although serious squeezes are rare today in diving, minor squeezes occur regularly. A squeeze occurs any time there is an air space either in, on, or attached to the body, where there is a pressure differential.

While the squeezes presented here do not cause fatal injuries, they can be painful and disorienting for the diver, and might cause panic leading to drowning or other injuries.

Mask Squeeze

In recreational diving, a sport diver can suffer a mask squeeze if he fails to equalize the pressure in his mask with the surrounding water pressure. Since the pressure on the outside of the mask is greater than the pressure inside, the diver must take steps to equalize the pressure. Equalizing this pressure is easy; the diver simply exhales a small amount of air through his nose. However, if the diver fails to do this and continues to descend, the small blood vessels in the eye may rupture. In most cases, the diver will feel discomfort before this ever occurs and take the necessary steps to prevent this.

Middle Ear Squeeze

In all diving, it is essential for the diver to be able to equalize the air pressure in his middle ear. Equalization normally

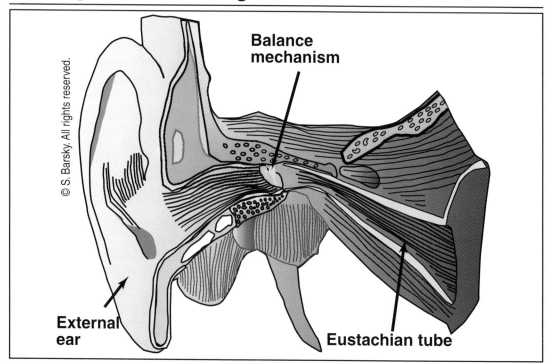

© S. Barsky. All rights reserved.

Balance mechanism

External ear

Eustachian tube

Fig. 4.1 It's not uncommon for divers to have difficulty equalizing the pressure in their ears.

takes place when air from the back of the throat is forced up through the Eustachian tube and into the middle ear space. If the tube is blocked, which can occur when the diver has a head cold, equalization is usually difficult or impossible.

When the diver has difficulty equalizing this pressure, the eardrum is forced inward due to the greater pressure on the outside, and is perceived as pain in the ear. If the diver continues to descend, the eardrum will eventually rupture, allowing cold water to enter the ear. This can lead to vertigo, nausea, and possibly panic, especially in an inexperienced diver.

A ruptured eardrum will usually heal in a few weeks time, but it's possible to develop an infection as a result. Divers who suffer from this type of injury should seek medical attention.

Sinus Squeeze

The sinuses are air spaces in the human skull that are lined with tissue. By having these spaces filled with air, the skull is lighter than it would be if made from solid bone.

When a diver submerges underwater, the air spaces of the sinuses equalize naturally with no effort on the diver's part, provided the diver has no sinus congestion due to allergies or a head cold. However, if the diver does have congestion, there is nothing he can do to equalize these spaces. If he continues to descend, blood and tissue will fill these voids in an attempt to equalize the pressure.

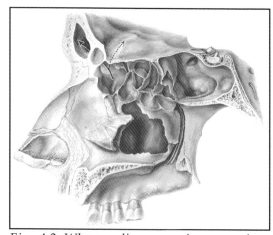

Fig. 4.2 When a diver experiences a sinus squeeze, there may be bleeding from the nose following a dive. (© Life-Art. All rights reserved.)

Contributing Factors in Diving Accidents

Nitrogen Narcosis

Nitrogen narcosis is a condition that affects most divers breathing compressed air at depths of 100 FSW and deeper. Different people have different reactions to nitrogen narcosis, but most people describe it as feeling as though they were intoxicated. While nitrogen narcosis will not cause death by itself, it has caused divers to have lapses in judgment and/or a failure to recognize when situations were becoming dangerous. Nitrogen narcosis may also affect the diver's perception of time.

The reason helium is used to replace nitrogen on deep dives by commercial and technical divers is that it does not cause the intoxication seen with breathing mixtures where nitrogen is the primary component.

Technical divers will frequently use gas mixtures containing helium, nitrogen, and oxygen. This type of mixture is commonly referred to as "tri-mix." Tri-mix is used because it is less expensive than using a straight helium-oxygen mixture.

In deep diving incidents where the diver is breathing compressed air, nitrogen narcosis should always be considered as a possible contributing factor.

Hypothermia

Hypothermia can be a problem in almost any diving environment where the water temperature is colder than the diver's body core temperature. Problems with heat loss underwater are dependent on a number of factors including the diver's body size and amount of subcutaneous fat, exercise level, type of breathing gas, and type of insulation worn by the diver. In warmer waters, although the diver may not subjectively feel cold, heat loss can still occur.

Hypothermia is defined as a significant drop in the core temperature of the body. The greater the drop, the more serious the effects. In extreme cases, people suffering from hypothermia can become unconscious.

While it is rare for a diver to die of hypothermia by itself, it can happen. However, in most cases, hypothermia leads to exhaustion or a loss of coordination or fine manipulation, which then results in an accident leading to death or drowning.

For sport divers making deep dives, heat loss through the lungs can be significant. As the air from the scuba tank expands, it cools down tremendously, which leads to increased heat loss from the lungs. Each time the diver inhales he must warm the cold air from the tank and each time he exhales, he loses heat.

Helium-oxygen gas mixtures have exceptionally high thermal conductivity. Recreational (technical) divers who regularly dive deep and use dry suits sometimes use a small separate gas cylinder filled with argon to inflate their dry suits to avoid the heat loss that would occur from introducing helium into their suits.

Recently, quantitative studies have been done on the subject and it is not clear that helium has a dramatic effect on respiratory heat loss until you reach the

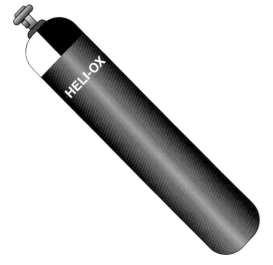

Fig. 4.3 Helium-oxygen mixtures (heli-ox) are used for deep diving by both technical and commercial divers.

deeper depths where commercial divers work. At equal depths, the respiratory heat loss breathing air is actually greater than the respiratory heat loss breathing an equivalent "heli-ox" mix. However, the thermal conductivity of helium when a diver is surrounded by the gas, for example in a saturation system, is important.

Helium becomes a much more serious respiratory problem on deeper dives. On commercial dives deeper than 600 FSW, respiratory heat loss is serious enough that supplemental breathing gas heaters are recommended. The simplest method for heating a commercial diver's breathing gas is to install a "T" fitting in the hot water hose that supplies the diver's suit, and use a small stream of hot water to supply a shroud that can be fitted to the breathing system on the helmet. This external hot water heat supply is sufficient to heat the diver's breathing gas to help maintain the diver's internal core temperature.

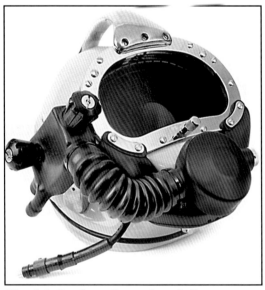

Fig. 4.4 On deep dives where helium-oxygen is used, a hot water shroud should be installed over the breathing system on the helmet to help heat the diver's breathing gas. (© Kirby Morgan Dive Systems, Inc. All rights reserved.)

High Breathing Resistance

Although most diving equipment available on the market today has excellent breathing characteristics, occasionally equipment does appear on the market that causes the diver to work hard just to breathe. In addition, equipment that normally works well may develop high breathing resistance due to a lack of maintenance or improper adjustment.

While one might suppose that resistance to inhalation would be the most important consideration in designing life support equipment, resistance to exhalation is generally considered more important. The amount of effort required to breathe underwater using a particular regulator or diving helmet is known as "work of breathing." Some equipment manufacturers maintain extremely sophisticated equipment for conducting their own tests.

The U.S. Navy and other organizations have developed standardized tests for underwater breathing apparatus at specific work loads. These tests are conducted using a special "breathing machine" and a hyperbaric chamber that simulates a diver breathing at specific work rates and at various depths. Results from these tests are analyzed against standards established by the Navy to determine whether a particular piece of equipment is performing at an acceptable level.

Some scuba retailers will have the facilities to service and adjust regulators using a device known as a "magnehelic gauge" to adjust the "cracking pressure" of a regulator. This is the point at which the regulator begins to flow air when the diver inhales. This is a simple but crude measure of a regulator's performance and nowhere near as accurate as tests conducted on a breathing machine. In addition, a magnehelic gauge will only measure inhalation resistance and does not measure exhalation effort at all.

Most forensic laboratories do not have

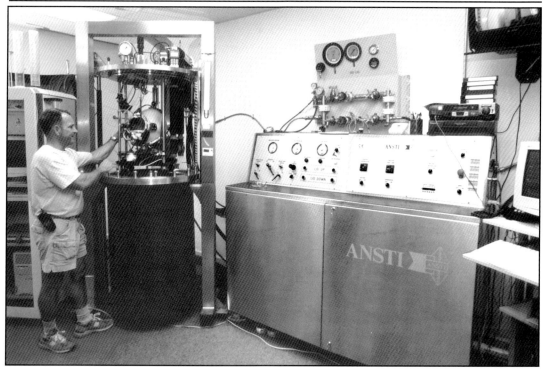

Fig. 4.5 Accurate tests of the performance of a regulator are only possible on a breathing machine like this one at the Dive Lab in Panama City, Florida.

the facilities to test regulators, but instead rely on outside laboratories when they need accurate information on the performance of a piece of gear. For example, in the past, the L.A. County Coroner's office would send any equipment involved in a diving accident to the UCLA Kinesiology lab for testing. The Naval Experimental Diving Unit in Panama City has also conducted testing for some law enforcement agencies from time to time and provides guidance for the U.S. Coast Guard in commercial diving investigations. Private laboratories are also available which can conduct these tests.

When breathing resistance is high, a diver working at even moderate work loads may find that he is unable to breathe at a comfortable level. When the diver cannot exchange a sufficient volume of breathing gas a situation occurs which is commonly referred to as "overbreathing" the regulator. This can lead to a feeling of suffocation which can cause panic.

The most extreme example of this has already been mentioned. Should a diver mistakenly open his tank valve only one quarter of a turn, at depth the diver will experience the sensation that his equipment has failed and he is not getting air. This type of situation occurs because divers are routinely trained to open the tank valve all the way and then close it one quarter turn. When people forget which way to open the valve, they close the valve all the way and then open it one quarter turn. Several fatalities have occurred as a result of this mistake.

Exhaustion

Diving can be easy to participate in, but it can also be a very physically demanding sport. Diving on a tropical reef in warm, shallow water with no current is something almost anyone in reasonable health can enjoy. Little equipment is required, and divers don't have to exert much physical effort.

Conversely, diving in cold water or where there are strong currents or high surf, is much more challenging. The work load of dressing into a thick wetsuit, donning a heavy tank and weights, and swimming on the surface to the descent point is high and can be quite fatiguing to someone who is not in good physical condition.

In most cases, even if the diver becomes exhausted, there are many things that he can do to rest and recover while still in the water. If the diver is underwater, the best thing that he can do is to simply stop all activity and just breathe for however long it takes for him to recover. If he is on the surface, it is a simple matter for a scuba diver to inflate his buoyancy compensator and rest on the surface.

A high number of scuba diving fatalities occur on the surface. The typical scenario involves a diver at the end of his dive who is swimming on the surface to return to the boat. Whether it is due to a current or his own poor physical condition, the diver becomes exhausted, stops swimming in a horizontal position, and

turns upright to get his head out of the water.

Once the diver is in a vertical position in the water, it becomes difficult for him to breathe for comfort. Two factors are at work here. First, if the diver is not positively buoyant, he is supporting the weight of his head and the top of his scuba tank out of the water. In most cases, this is at least 15 pounds of weight that he is struggling to lift above the surface. In addition, when the diver is vertical in the water, there is greater water pressure on the chest, making it difficult to inhale.

A number of deaths have occurred in these circumstances. Whether these deaths were primarily due to exhaustion and subsequent drowning, or whether they were caused by an underlying medical condition cannot always be determined. (See the section on interpreting the autopsy in the last chapter of the book.)

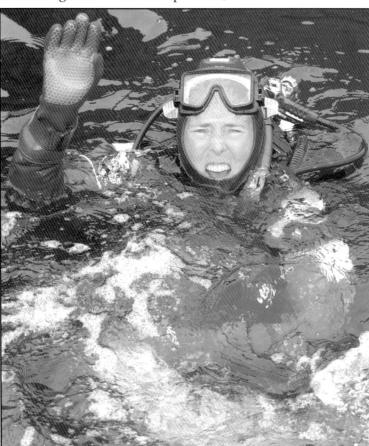

Fig. 4.6 A diver who is vertical in the water and treading water will quickly become exhausted.

Carotid Sinus Reflex

The carotid arteries are two blood vessels that run along either side of your neck to provide the primary blood supply and oxygen to the brain. These vessels must never be pinched off or unconsciousness will occur.

Some types of diving gear, such as the neck seals on dry suits and helmets, can place pressure on the carotid arteries, if the seals are not properly adjusted prior to use. Obviously, anything that would cause a diver to pass out underwater is highly undesirable. Fortunately, it's a simple matter to adjust these pieces of equipment prior to diving.

The role of this reflex in diving accidents may be more theoretical than real, but it is a factor of which you should be cognizant.

Hyperthermia

Hyperthermia occurs when a person's core temperature is raised above the normal temperature. Although this is an unusual situation to occur in diving, it can happen. Hyperthermia is especially serious when it occurs underwater because the normal mechanism by which a person would cool down in air, i.e., through evaporative cooling from perspiration, is totally ineffective underwater.

Hyperthermia in the natural environment is rare, but commercial and professional divers sometimes find themselves in situations where hyperthermia is a distinct possibility. For example, commercial divers sometimes must enter closed environments where the water has been deliberately heated, such as a water tank on a oil drilling rig or the cooling pond in a nuclear reactor. Divers who use dry suits to dive in polluted waters sometimes dive in situations where there can be an extreme build-up of heat inside their suit.

In these situations, steps must be taken to cool the diver properly to avoid overheating. If this is not done, an adverse outcome can result. Divers have used cooling vests and special "tube" suits that circulate cooling water around their bodies to maintain a normal core temperature.

Hypoxia

Hypoxia is the medical term that means "low oxygen." Although it is rare for a sport diver to suffer from hypoxia, it is a common cause of rebreather diving accidents, and an occasional cause of commercial diving accidents.

Divers using semi-closed circuit rebreathers are especially susceptible to hypoxic incidents. It is possible with this type of system to consume more oxygen than the system supplies, particularly at high work loads and with divers who are in good physical condition. In a situation where the semi-closed circuit rebreather is functioning properly, but the diver fails to turn on the breathing gas and does not have an oxygen monitoring system, all of the oxygen in the breathing bags may be consumed.

Hypoxia can occur in a commercial diving accident if the diver is supplied with a gas mixture containing an inadequate amount of oxygen for the depth at which he is working. Although this type of accident is rare, it can occur.

In some cases, a pathologist may not recognize hypoxia as the underlying cause of death in a rebreather diving incident and may simply assign the cause of death as drowning, since once the diver loses consciousness he may lose the mouthpiece and drown.

Hyperoxia

Hyperoxia is a situation that occurs when the partial pressure of oxygen in the breathing gas mixture is too high. In a mixture of gases, each gas exerts a pressure, known as its partial pressure, independent of the other gases in the mix.

Under normal circumstances, the air we breathe contains approximately 20% oxygen and 79% nitrogen at the surface. As the diver descends in the water column, the partial pressure of each gas in the breathing mixture increases. As the partial pressure of oxygen increases beyond 1.4-1.6 atmospheres absolute (ATA) the risk of an oxygen induced seizure increases. The higher the partial pressure of oxygen, the shorter the exposure can be prior to the onset of a generalized "fit." Unless the diver is equipped with special equipment, a convulsion underwater may lead to drowning.

For dives deeper than 200 feet, the breathing gas mixture is normally something other than compressed air. In most cases, the diver will breathe a mixture of helium and oxygen. The helium is used to replace the nitrogen, which can cause narcosis at depths below 100 feet. Technical divers, professional divers, and commercial divers may use gas mixtures containing very low percentages of oxygen during the deep portions of their dives.

Pure oxygen may be used underwater in certain situations, but this is uncommon in most circumstances. The toxicity of pure oxygen (O_2) limits its use to depths less than 20-25 FSW.

Military divers use pure oxygen in fully closed-circuit rebreathers used for clandestine purposes because they emit no bubbles. Scientific divers have also used pure oxygen for capturing creatures like sea otters, that might be alerted to a diver's presence by the bubbles released by ordinary scuba equipment.

Technical diving accidents have occurred where a diver has mistakenly used an oxygen rich decompression mixture on the bottom, at a depth beyond where breathing such a mixture is safe. Similar accidents have occurred in the commercial diving industry.

Carbon Dioxide "Poisoning" (CO_2)

Carbon dioxide is a by-product of respiration that is produced as our body consumes some of the oxygen that we inhale with each breath of air that we take. The normal amount of oxygen in air when we inhale is approximately 20%. When we breathe out, we exhale about 16% oxygen and 4% carbon dioxide.

As we produce carbon dioxide in our bodies, it serves to activate the trigger mechanism that causes us to breathe. Obviously, a bit of carbon dioxide is a good thing. However, too much carbon dioxide in the breathing gas supply can overstimulate the breathing mechanism, leaving the diver feeling as though he cannot get enough air. Since carbon dioxide is odorless and has only a slightly acidic taste, a diver may be completely unaware of a build-up of this gas until it is too late.

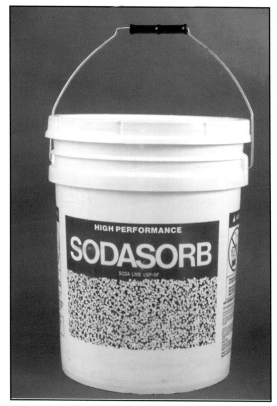

Fig. 4.7 Chemical absorbents such as Sodasorb® are used in rebreathers to remove the carbon dioxide from the breathing loop.

Carbon dioxide "poisoning" is rarely a contributing factor in a diving accident involving open circuit scuba, or most commercial diving equipment, but may be an important factor in a rebreather diving accident. Most open circuit diving equipment today is very good at reducing the amount of carbon dioxide that the diver may breathe.

Rebreathers always include some mechanism for removing carbon dioxide from the breathing "loop." The most common method for cleansing the carbon dioxide from the system is to use a chemical "absorbent." This material undergoes a chemical reaction that removes the carbon dioxide and produces heat and moisture as by-products of this change. The absorbent is normally located in a plastic container called a "scrubber," which is usually a cylinder with the chemical absorbent inside, integrated into the breathing system. The most common chemical used in the scrubber is baralyme, which is sold under commercial names, such as Sodasorb®. Divers may also refer to this chemical as the "scrubber" as well.

Carbon dioxide "poisoning" can occur in a rebreather in several ways. First, if the diver completely fails to load the absorbent into the scrubber canister, there will be nothing to absorb carbon dioxide and it will build up rapidly in the system. Another way this could happen is if the diver fails to fill the absorbent canister properly, and the breathing gas does not pass through the absorbent but flows through "channels" in the canister where it does not come into contact with the absorbent. This problem is known as "channeling." Still a third problem that may occur is if the absorbent is used past the time at which it operates correctly, so that it is no longer effective in absorbing CO_2.

Many years ago, when the U.S. Navy was conducting the SeaLab III experiment off the coast of California at San Clemente island, the Navy blamed the death of one

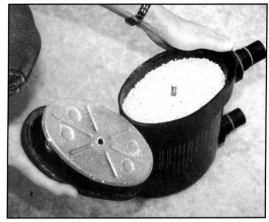

Fig. 4.8 Rebreather scrubber cannisters must be carefully sealed to prevent water from entering the breathing circuit.

of the divers on the failure to load carbon dioxide absorbent into the diver's breathing gear. Subsequent information from Dr. John Rawlins, who examined the diver's rebreather, discounts this explanation, although such an incident surely would have been fatal in 600 FSW.

Drowning

Drowning is said to be the most common cause of death in a diving accident, however you should never automatically assume that just because an autopsy lists the cause of death as drowning that the coroner is correct. In many rural areas, it is not uncommon for the authorities to make the assumption, "he's wet, he's dead, he drowned."

Unless the coroner is knowledgeable about diving accident victims, he may not know what to look for or what he is looking at. Autopsies performed on diving accident victims must be performed in a specific manner to detect problems such as air embolism, a type of lung over-pressure injury. If an air embolism is suspected, the heart can be opened with water in the pericardial sac so that air bubbles can be more easily detected.

Obviously, drownings also occur underwater, too. One typical scenario is the diver who is overweighted or has failed to establish neutral buoyancy during a deep dive in low visibility. In this situation, the diver is usually near the end of his dive and low on air. As the diver begins to ascend, he looks up as he has been trained to do, but either fails to watch his dive computer or may be in dark water with no visible reference. The diver kicks and kicks but without proper buoyancy control makes no progress towards the surface. He may be just a few inches or feet off the bottom, stirring up clouds of silt when he finally runs out of air or drains the tank past the point where it can supply sufficient air pressure. If the diver fails to establish positive buoyancy to ascend, he will drown.

At deeper depths, where wetsuit compression may be extreme (usually at depths of 100 feet or greater) even if the diver drops his belt he may have insufficient buoyancy to leave the bottom if no air has been added to the buoyancy compensator. In addition, some of the newer high-pressure cylinders, particularly those used in technical diving, have sufficient negative buoyancy that some divers do not even wear a weight belt. In these cases, they are entirely dependent on the buoyancy of their dry suit and/or buoyancy compensator to help them establish positive buoyancy.

When a diver drowns he aspirates (breathes into the lungs) some water. Until recently, it was believed that an individual could drown without aspirating. However, newer information strongly suggests that these so called "dry drownings" cannot occur, and thus, the diagnosis of drowning in a diver without aspiration must be re-examined by the accident investigator very carefully, and other causes of death must be looked for assiduously.

Lung Over-Pressure Accidents

There are several different types of lung over-pressure accidents, most of which are not immediately fatal. In a lung over-pressure incident, the diver must be breathing compressed air underwater at the start of the incident. If the diver holds his breath and swims rapidly to the surface, the lung tissues can rupture as the compressed air in them expands as the water pressure decreases.

The usual types of lung injuries include arterial gas embolism (AGE) and mediastinal emphysema. Less common injuries are subcutaneous emphysema and pneumothorax.

In the case of an arterial gas embolism, the small air sacs in the lungs known as the "alveoli" rupture. Air then can be introduced into the blood stream, which can then go to the brain and block the flow of blood. In serious cases, this can cause death very quickly, but there have been many cases where victims have survived an AGE and completely recovered when they have received rapid first aid and recompression therapy. This involves administering 100% oxygen. However, for definitive treatment, the victim will almost always be treated in a hyperbaric chamber.

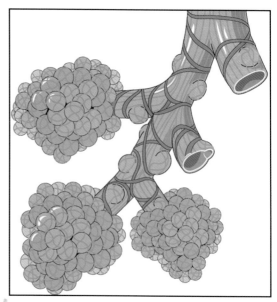

Fig. 4.9 The alveoli are delicate and can be damaged by only a slight pressure differential. *(© Life-Art. All rights reserved.)*

> **Risk Recognition for Divers and Diving Professionals**
>
> The law has made it very clear, whenever you are providing equipment that has a potential to cause injury or death, you must provide sufficiently clear warnings regarding these hazards. For a manufacturer in the diving industry, this means that not only must the equipment itself carry sufficient warnings, but there must also be information in the manuals that accompany the equipment about these risks.
>
> Likewise, if you are a diving equipment retailer, you must ensure that all of the original product labeling and warnings are given to any customer who buys a given piece of gear. It is imperative that all of the literature, labels, and hang tags you received from the manufacturer are delivered to the end user.

Symptoms of AGE include loss of consciousness, convulsions, paralysis, blindness, and chest pain.

In a pneumothorax, the lung wall ruptures and air enters the chest cavity, collapsing the lung. This is a serious injury, but fortunately is usually not fatal by itself.

In mediastinal emphysema air escapes from the lungs and is trapped in the tissues of the chest. If it is noticeable under the skin, (usually near the neck) it is called subcutaneous emphysema.

Carbon Monoxide Poisoning

Carbon monoxide (CO) is a waste gas that is normally produced as a by-product of an internal combustion engine. The gas is colorless, odorless, and tasteless, but extremely toxic.

Carbon monoxide has a tremendous affinity for hemoglobin, the chemical in red blood cells that transports oxygen throughout the body. When carbon monoxide bonds with hemoglobin it is extremely difficult to break this bond.

The most common situation where a diver may be exposed to carbon monoxide poisoning is when an air compressor intake is placed too close to the exhaust from the gasoline or diesel engine used to "drive" the compressor. Whether the carbon monoxide is fed into a compressed gas cylinder which is used by a diver at some later date, or delivered to a diver breathing compressed air from a hose

from the surface, the results are the same. The diver can pass out with little or no warning that there is any problem.

Carbon monoxide poisoning can also occur as a result of breathing air from an improperly operating, or improperly lubricated, air compressor, even if the power source used to drive the compressor is an electric motor. If the compressor is not properly maintained, it may generate carbon monoxide as previously mentioned. One of the authors personally witnessed this type of event aboard a dive boat in Southern California. One diver passed out and several others came perilously close to unconsciousness after breathing from tanks filled by an old and poorly operating compressor on the vessel.

Accidents Involving Boats

When divers and boats must share the same space, there is always a chance that accidental encounters will take place. This happens with both recreational and commercial divers.

In sport diving, the size of the boat and how the boat strikes the diver will determine the nature and extent of the injury. Divers have been knocked unconscious and drowned when the hull of even a small boat has hit their heads. The most gruesome type of injury occurs when a turning propeller strikes a diver. Even the propeller of a small boat can cause a serious or fatal injury. When the propeller of a large boat strikes a diver, this may lead to a loss of a limb and is often fatal.

When propellers strike divers, death may result due to extensive bleeding or from direct trauma. In one case, a diver was struck by a boat that took off the top of the diver's head.

Some encounters between divers and boats take place because divers fail to fly the proper flag to indicate their presence in the water. However, in many cases, boat operators have either failed to see the flag, ignored the flag, or not understood what the flag meant.

Decompression Sickness

Air is a mixture of primarily two gases, nitrogen and oxygen. Our bodies consume oxygen, but nitrogen is essentially an "inert" gas that is absorbed by the body but not used. When we are at sea level, the nitrogen in our bodies is in equilibrium with the surrounding pressure.

When a diver breathing compressed air goes underwater, the pressure on his body increases. To be able to breathe, the pressure in the diver's lungs must equal the pressure surrounding him.

In scuba diving, the regulator supplies compressed air to the diver's lungs at a pressure exactly equal to the surrounding (ambient) pressure. With each breath the diver takes, he absorbs additional nitrogen to establish a new equilibrium. This

nitrogen is absorbed through the lungs and into the blood stream up to the point of a new equilibrium. The longer the diver stays underwater, or the deeper he dives, the more nitrogen he absorbs.

"Decompression sickness" is the term used to refer to the signs and symptoms that may occur in a diver following a dive due to the evolution of a gas phase (bubbles) that transpires when pressure surrounding the diver is decreased and a supersaturated state in the body occurs. Bubbles then form in the tissues and it is these bubbles that cause DCS. The type and severity of DCS depends largely upon the quantity and location of the bubbles that arise.

To avoid suffering from decompression sickness, divers either use decompression tables or a dive computer. Decompression tables are a set of calculations that are used in conjunction with a watch and depth gauge to calculate allowable bottom time. These calculations are based upon testing conducted by the U.S. Navy or other private organizations.

Today, most divers use a dive computer to calculate their bottom time and depth. The dive computer automatically calculates bottom time and depth every few seconds and provides the diver with a display of his remaining allowable dive time at any given depth. Most computers will also record other factors such as water temperature and some will even

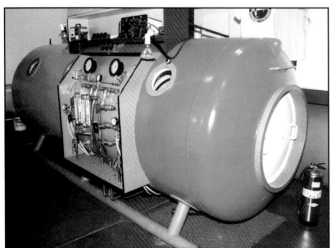

Fig. 4.10 In most areas where there is a high level of diving activity, you'll find a hyperbaric chamber to treat decompression sickness. This chamber is located in Pacific Grove, near Monterey, California.

monitor the diver's breathing rate. More sophisticated computers will compare the amount of air remaining in the diver's tank to his bottom time to determine which is the more limiting factor at any given time. The "downloadable" dive computer is the ultimate "black box" for the dive accident investigator.

Diving physicians and chamber operators may refer to Type I or Type II decompression sickness. Type I decompression sickness involves pain only. The symptoms are usually joint pain, and this is considered a less "serious" form of decompression sickness.

Type II decompression sickness refers to cases where there is neurological involvement. This can lead to paralysis, loss of bladder control, or other serious symptoms.

In any case of decompression sickness it usually is beneficial to get the victim on 100% oxygen as soon as possible. Every effort must be made to get the victim to a

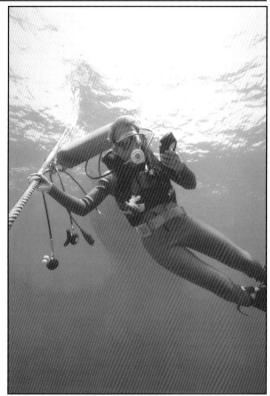

Fig. 4.12 It is considered routine to complete a precautionary decompression stop or "safety stop" at the end of each sport dive. The typical stop is three to five minutes at a depth of 10-15 feet.

decompression chamber immediately.

In many cases of decompression sickness there will be a clear cut violation of the dive tables or a dive computer. However, divers have experienced what is known as an "undeserved hit," i.e., where decompression sickness occurs for no obvious reason.

Commercial and technical divers who use gas mixtures other than air, such as helium and oxygen, or "tri-mix" containing helium, oxygen, and nitrogen, can also suffer decompression sickness. Due to the depths at which they dive, and their extended bottom times, which usually far exceed those of recreational divers, their cases of decompression sickness may be more serious.

It is uncommon for decompression sickness to cause a fatality, but it can occur. Most fatal decompression accidents

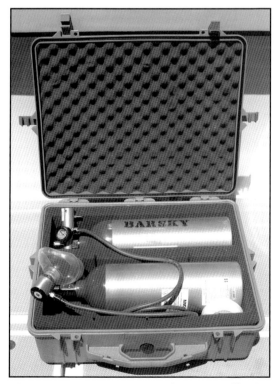

Fig. 4.11 Pure oxygen is the most effective first aid treatment for a diver suffering from decompression sickness.

occur in cases where the diver has an extreme decompression obligation and has missed all or part of his decompression. A double fatality occurred in this way that is well documented in the book, *The Last Dive*, written by Bernie Chowdhury.

Decompression sickness can also occur when a diver travels to altitude, either on land or in an airplane, following a dive or series of dives, which under ordinary circumstances might pose no problems. The reduced pressure at altitude allows what otherwise might be "silent" bubbles in the blood stream to grow to a size that causes decompression sickness.

The current recommendation of the Divers Alert Network (DAN), a non-profit divers' medical and health research organization, is that divers should wait a minimum of 12 hours following their last dive before flying in a commercial (pressurized) aircraft. If the diver has made multiple dives over a series of days, a longer interval (24 hours) is recommended. Many dive computers provide calculations based on the algorithm they use as to when it is theoretically "safe" to fly following diving. However, it is never possible to assure that all divers using

these devices will be able to fly without incident.

Helmet Squeeze

In commercial diving, a serious squeeze can occur if the diver is using surface-supplied gear and the topside air supply is lost. Under normal circumstances, a one-way (non-return) valve is supposed to be installed between the diver's helmet and supply hose. Both industry standards and government standards require this device.

If the air supply is lost and the valve is operating properly, the valve immediately closes preventing any loss of pressure from the helmet. However, if the valve is missing, defective, or otherwise non-functional, all of the air in the helmet will vent up the hose and the diver's body will be "squeezed" to attempt to fill the space inside the helmet. This can be fatal. While helmet squeezes are rare today, a serious helmet squeeze occurred in the Gulf of Mexico during the mid-1980s. A diver working in shallow water jumped off a barge and failed to check to see if the compressor was running. Although there was some air in the volume tank,

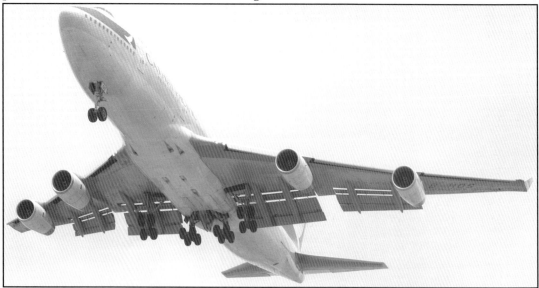

Fig. 4.13 The minimum recommended interval that sport divers should wait following diving in a pressurized aircraft is 12 hours. If the diver has been engaged in multiple days of diving, decompression or saturation diving, it is recommended that the diver wait for 24 hours before flying.

Case History – Recreational Divers

A group of divers signed up for a dive at a tropical resort famous for its swift currents. Under these conditions, most dives are conducted as "drift dives," where the boat is not anchored, but follows the divers by tracking their bubbles as the divers drift with the currents. Since it is extremely difficult to swim against a current of more than one knot in speed, this is the easiest way to dive under these conditions. The divers can cover a lot of ground without expending much effort.

The divers were diving out of a small boat that carried eight divers plus a divemaster. One of the buddy teams aboard the boat was a single father with his teenage son, neither of whom were experienced divers.

When the group got down to the bottom, the current was quite strong, and flowing out towards sea. The divemaster was having a difficult time keeping the group together, as some of the divers did not seem to realize the speed of the current. When one diver appeared to be having some difficulty with his buoyancy, the divemaster went to his aid and when he turned to check on the rest of the group, the man and his teenage son had disappeared.

At that point, the divemaster sent the remainder of the divers to the surface and started to search for the lost dive team. As he neared the drop-off, where the reef ended in a vertical face, he realized that the man and his son had probably been swept out towards sea and without a nearby bottom for reference, were probably drifting much deeper than the top of the reef, which was at 80 FSW.

Reaching the end of the reef, the divemaster continued out into the blue water of the open channel and began to descend, searching for the missing divers. He found them at a depth of 165 FSW, both of them seemingly unaware of the danger they were in. Presumably, they were suffering from the effects of nitrogen narcosis and were oblivious to their situation.

The divemaster brought the man and his son up successfully. All three were immediately rushed to the closest decompression chamber, where they underwent a prophylactic decompression treatment, despite the fact they had no symptoms. The man, his son, and the divemaster exited the chamber without further incident. This could have been an extremely serious accident if the divemaster had not located the man and his son.

which gave the diver the false impression that he had adequate breathing gas, the air quickly ran out. As the diver made a rapid descent, the air in the helmet was depleted. The non-return valve in the helmet failed, but fortunately one of the topside tenders caught the diver's hose and stopped his descent. Even so, the diver stopped breathing, and suffered massive hemorrhage of the blood vessels in his eyes. The diver was successfully resuscitated and fully recovered, but the whites of his eyes were totally red for almost two months after the incident.

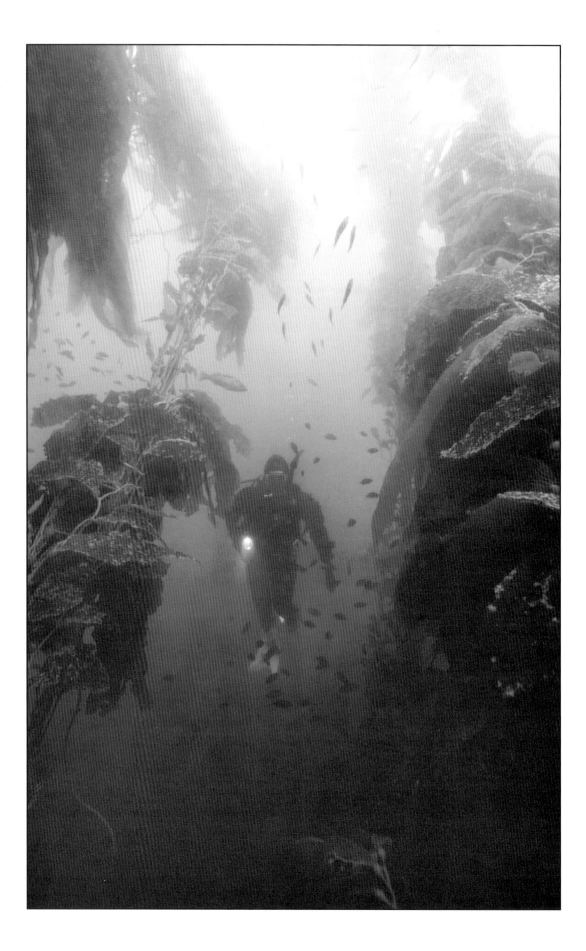

Chapter 5
Talents and Characteristics of the Dive Accident Investigator

The successful diving accident investigator needs a variety of skills and traits to do the job properly. Above all, he needs to be a knowledgeable, competent diver, a writer, and a photographer, so that he can put together a cogent and effective report. He must have good organizational skills, be capable of critical thinking, and have dogged determination to ferret out information.

It also helps to have a sympathetic personality so that people will be willing to talk to you. Finally, a good investigator always has an open mind and does not form or express opinions, but deals only in facts. Let's take an in-depth look at each of these skills and characteristics so you will understand how to develop them in yourself.

Diving Experience and Knowledge

Unless you have broad and varied diving experience, it's unlikely you will be a good diving accident investigator. There is no way that you can appreciate the problems that a diving instructor might experience while training students on a night dive unless you have done this type of dive yourself.

While it's not essential for you to be a diving instructor, it is crucial that you be intimately familiar with the instructional and training standards followed by the sport diver training agencies. Similarly, if you are going to investigate commer-

cial diving accidents, you need to have a background and experience in commercial diving.

Without extensive diving experience and knowledge, it's impossible to visualize an accident scenario and understand what took place, or to know whether the incident someone relates to you is plausible or not. Without appropriate experience it is difficult or impossible to see what information is missing from the data that has already been collected. If you aren't familiar with the fact that the saturation technician should keep a log of all items locked in and out of the diving system, it is unlikely that you will ask to see this document.

Technical Knowledge of Dive Gear

With the wide range of diving equipment available today, it's unrealistic to expect any one person to know how each piece of diving equipment works. However, the competent dive accident investigator will have at least basic familiarity with each different class of equipment, from regulators to dive computers. You need to understand the technical concepts and principles behind the equipment, rather than have an end user's knowledge of the functional characteristics of each dive computer on the market. If you understand the principles of how the gear operates, you can sort out the fine details from owners' and shop manuals.

Experienced investigators have a knowledge of the history of the industry so that they usually know at least some of the trends and thinking that went into the development of a piece of equipment. This is especially useful when you run into older pieces of equipment during the course of your investigation.

Another crucial aspect of being a successful investigator is having sufficient industry contacts who can fill in any gaps in your knowledge. No one person knows everything there is to know about diving, so it's important to have contacts who can educate you in any areas where you might be lacking information. For example, if you need information on the intricacies of a dive computer, there's no substitute for being able to call an engineer who worked on its development to ask him any technical questions you might need answered.

It is also helpful to have or develop contacts with local law enforcement agencies, the Coast Guard, and other organizations that may provide useful information for your investigation.

Investigators Must Be Organized

Most recreational diving accidents will involve a large number of people since diving is a social sport and often takes place aboard charter boats. In addition, multiple agencies usually respond when an accident occurs. For this reason, there is usually a large amount of information collected during an accident investigation and good organization is critical.

If you are investigating an accident that took place at a remote location and you must travel, your investigation will require even more organization. You will need to coordinate with all of the various parties involved to make the most efficient use of your time while you are on the road.

Frequently, it's also helpful if your investigation follows a logical sequence so that you collect certain information and interviews before others. For example, if you are not familiar with the dive site and it has any unusual features, it may be quite helpful to inspect the site prior to conducting any of the interviews, so you

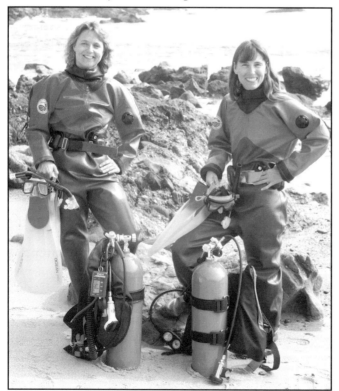

Fig. 5.1 A good diving investigator is familiar with the history of the industry and can readily recognize and identify equipment from different time periods. Can you put a date on the equipment in this photo?

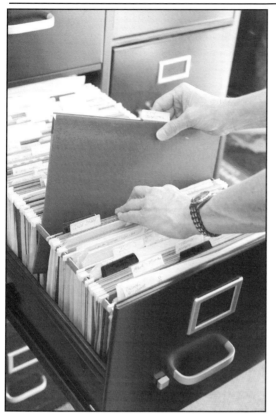

Fig. 5.2 Diving accident investigators must be highly organized.

have a better understanding of what took place.

Part of being organized also entails making sure that you have all of the materials on hand that you will need to conduct your investigation. It's a good practice to prepare a detailed checklist of the items that you normally use. The list can be modified for specific cases.

Commercial diving accidents may also involve a large number of people, since most commercial diving operations involve teams of divers. When an accident takes place aboard a barge or drilling rig, there may be many witnesses who have knowledge about the accident and what took place.

Your Report is the Product of Your Investigation

At the end of the day, your report is the end product of your investigation, and it is how your work will be judged. It doesn't matter how good a job you have done collecting information. If you cannot communicate your findings in a clear and logical manner, you will not be considered an effective investigator.

Although some people have natural writing ability, for most people, writing is a learned skill. Almost everyone can learn to write in a straightforward, objective manner.

Your report must also be developed in a logical sequence. The report should include a detailed chronology of events, a description of the site, and a synopsis of what took place. Individual interviews should be in the order in which those involved had contact with the victim.

Risk Recognition for Divers and Diving Professionals

Divers frequently modify their equipment to improve the fit or performance of a particular item. In most cases, these modifications are harmless, but in some circumstances, these changes can lead to accidents.

Commercial divers in particular frequently modify their equipment to make it fit their needs. Modifications to diving helmets are particularly risky and have resulted in diving accidents.

Recreational divers also use gear in ways the manufacturer did not intend. One of the most extreme examples, is the use of one of the most popular types of semi-closed circuit rebreathers. Shortly after the product became available, technical divers discovered that by using the rebreather with gas mixtures other than those originally intended, dives could be made to great depths. This demands that the diver make the correct partial pressure calculations, carry sufficient gas, and plan his decompression properly. This is an extreme example of a situation that carries a high potential for an accident.

Very frequently, accurate medical diagnoses will depend on the exact sequence of events. It is therefore extremely important to obtain a complete and precise description of the sequence of events. In this regard, having a thorough working knowledge of the various injuries that can befall a diver becomes very useful. All too often, coroner's reports are incorrect because the critical sequence of the events is not available at the time of autopsy.

Even though your computer will undoubtedly have a spelling and grammar checker, it's still important to have someone else read your report for content. If nothing else, you want to be sure that your report is clear. Appropriate grammar is essential and the report must be written in an unambiguous style that is not open to interpretation.

Photographs and Illustrations Make Reports More Interesting

With today's automatic digital cameras, there's no reason for a report not to include clear, well exposed photographs.

With the addition of a scanner, copies of documents, nautical charts, and other items are also easily included.

The photographs in your report should properly illustrate the details that you want them to show. Most cameras today can be used in a macro mode that will allow you to capture the small details of the equipment, such as serial numbers, which should also be included in the text of the report.

Investigators Must be Critical Thinkers

To be an effective investigator you must be capable of seeing beyond the immediate information that has been provided to you. You must understand and interpret actions and evidence in light of their implications in a particular diving situation.

A good diving accident investigator is able to look at a situation and see not only what is there, but more importantly, what might be missing. The missing equipment, information, or procedures may be the key to why the accident took place.

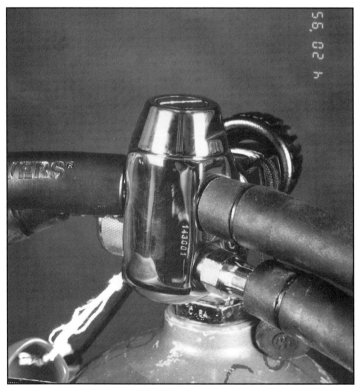

Fig. 5.3 Good clear photographs will make your report more interesting and complete.

Another key skill in dive accident investigation is the ability to look at a piece of equipment or situation and understand what you're seeing. If you don't know the equipment well enough, you may not realize if a particular piece is broken or improperly assembled.

Investigators Must be Tenacious

Diving accident investigators must develop an "ice-pick mentality," i.e., they must be highly focused on their job. It's often difficult to get certain documents and unless you are dogged in your determination, your report may be lacking in critical information. Witnesses are sometimes reluctant to talk or don't want to spend the time to meet. If you are not persistent you may miss information that might change your report.

Although you may be anxious to conclude your investigation and complete your report, don't be afraid to go back and revisit a site, re-interview a witness, or review a document. Many times, after you've completed an interview, or have interviewed a new witness, some new question or fact will arise that must be verified.

Don't be afraid to be like "Columbo," the detective from the old television program who always went back with "just one more question."

Make the effort to interview as many of the people as possible who might have any information regarding the incident. In certain cases, it's possible for a person to have seen something that nobody else may have seen that would cast the case in a different light.

Investigators Must Be Personable

The best investigators are extremely personable and have "magnetic" personalities. They are able to gather information easily because people want to talk to them and share information with them. Collecting information through intimidation or bullying people is usually not as effective as gathering information from people who feel comfortable with you and do not perceive you as a threat.

Good Investigators Have No Opinion

Unless you are a police officer investigating a homicide, or an expert witness working for an attorney, there is usually no place for a personal opinion in most dive accident investigations. Your job as an investigator is to gather the facts and report them. This is equally true for investigators who are working for insurance companies, attorneys, or civil agencies.

Investigators Must Be Discreet

A good investigator must be a master of both discretion and diplomacy, and must fully understand that the information that he collects is considered confidential and not to be shared with friends or casual acquaintances.

Careless bragging about what you know about a case could jeopardize its final outcome as well as your future as an investigator. Be discreet about what you know unless you have been authorized to discuss the issues surrounding the case with a particular person. If people quiz you about the case, and have no authority to have access to the information that you possess, be polite but change the subject. If you are pressured to divulge information by someone who has no right to it, explain to them in a courteous manner that you are not authorized to share the information that you hold.

This is particularly true for medical information you may gather. New laws concerning unauthorized disclosure of medical records are associated with large fines and even jail terms for unauthorized distribution of this data.

Case History – Introductory Diving Course

A diving instructor was working at a popular tropical resort destination that sees large numbers of tourists that have no experience in scuba diving. In an attempt to entice some of these visitors into taking scuba lessons, the resort offers low cost resort courses and discover scuba experiences that do not provide a full scuba certification, but allow a person to dive in shallow water under the direct supervision of an instructor.

On the day of this particular accident, the instructor was assigned to take a group of eleven resort trained tourists out for a dive on a shallow reef in 12 feet of water. The instructor was accompanied by a boat captain who ran the boat, but there was no divemaster or assistant instructor to help the instructor who had more non-certified divers than his training agency allowed him to supervise at one time in open water.

The dive itself went smoothly, but at the end of the dive, the instructor was uncertain about how to safely ascend with all of the divers at once. Instead, he brought up several of the novices at a time, leaving others on the bottom. When the instructor descended the last time to bring up the remaining three divers, he immediately noticed that one of them, a woman, was missing. After bringing the other divers to the surface, he returned to the bottom to search for the lost diver. After thirty minutes of searching, he found the woman unconscious on the bottom, with no air remaining in her tank. Although the instructor initiated CPR and medical evacuation procedures were initiated, all attempts to resuscitate the woman were unsuccessful.

This case was a clear violation of training standards. The instructor not only had more students in the water than his agency allowed, but also left a non-certified diver alone on the bottom.

Although clear standards violations were evident in this case, as a neutral party, the investigator provides only the facts of the accident. Unless specifically asked for an analysis, the investigator will normally provide no opinion on whether standards have been violated.

Notes:

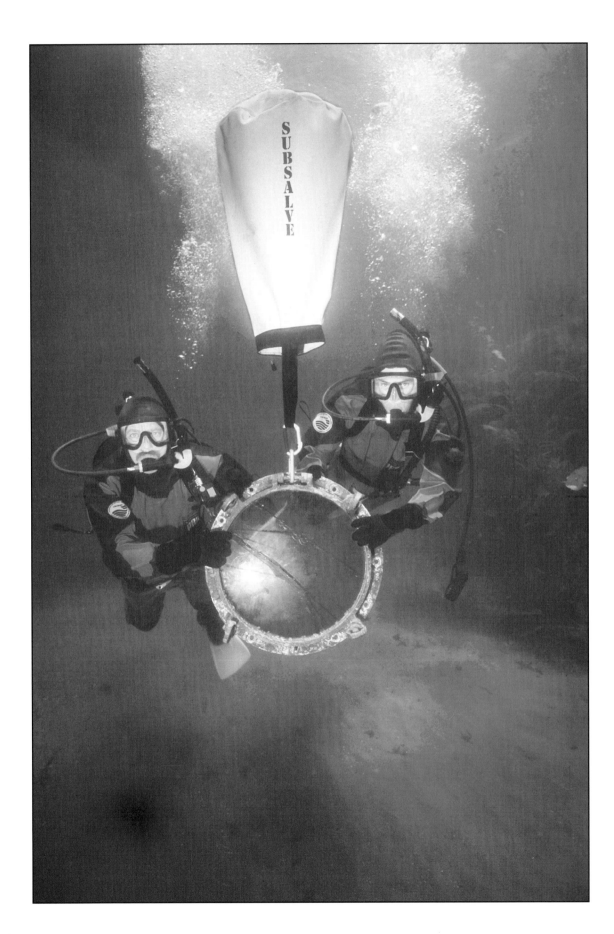

Chapter 6
The Tools of the Dive Accident Investigator

In any investigation of a diving accident, your single most important tool will be your mind. To be a successful investigator, you must continually be considering all the possibilities and implications of each piece of information that you collect. If you do not have an inquisitive nature, you must learn to develop one. It is critical for you to be open minded about the validity of decisions and opinions made by prior investigators if you have access to their reports. Your analysis must be independent of their conclusions.

Aside from your mind, there are a number of tools that you will need, no matter what type of investigation you are conducting. You won't need every tool for every investigation, but some of them will be indispensable in all cases. The most important items that you will need include the following:

- Film or Digital camera and/or video with underwater housing
- Laptop with modem and removable storage media
- Handheld organizer with computer interface and keyboard
- Color inkjet or laser printer
- Flatbed scanner
- Charts and or maps of the accident site and related points of interest (hospitals, fire stations, etc.)
- Fiberglass measuring tape (50 feet long)
- Voice recorder

- Magnifying glass
- Handheld GPS
- Oxygen analyzer
- Chalk

If you are required to submit certain items as part of your report, such as tape recorded interviews or photographs of witnesses, be sure to take back-up systems for any critical equipment. Don't take one micro-cassette recorder, take two. Don't take one camera, take two. Both pieces of gear don't need to be of the same quality, but they must both function and interface with the rest of your equipment easily.

Digital Camera and/or Video

To record photographic images of sites, equipment, and people, a digital still or video camera is essential. There may be some situations where you will want to use film, but for most applications, digital is preferable. Digital is faster and over the long haul it's cheaper, and the cameras tend to be quite compact.

Although there has been some legal discussion in Federal Court over the admissibility of digital images, this should not be a problem in most investigations. Check with the attorneys with whom you work if there is any doubt. Conventional cameras that use film have a number of advantages over video, but film cameras are being used less and less.

The current advantages to using con-

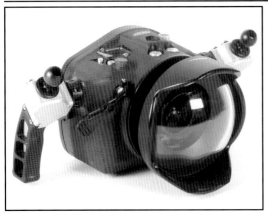

Fig. 6.1 Digital cameras provide immediate confirmation of your results. This underwater housing fits a Nikon digital camera.

ventional film are:

• Film cameras tend to be less expensive to purchase than comparable digital cameras

• Digital cameras tend to be more sensitive to extremes of heat and humidity

• If you need to blow photographs up to poster size, film may be a better choice, unless you own a professional quality digital camera with a resolution above 6 megapixels

Digital cameras, both those that produce only stills and those that produce video and still frames, are often a better choice for the dive accident investigator than a film camera. Perhaps the biggest advantage for an investigator working on a case in a remote area is the fact that you can instantly see your results in the camera, or download them to your laptop for viewing an enlarged version. This eliminates the possibility that you shot a poor exposure, didn't load film properly, the film was damaged, the lab misprocessed the film, you can't find a lab, you don't have the time to go to a lab, etc. There is no substitute for instant results.

Virtually all digital video cameras now have the capability to interface directly with a computer so that you can grab individual frames to make prints. "Frame grabs" are the least preferred

method of producing a print from a video camera due to their low resolution.

Many video cameras can now also shoot individual still images. However, the still photos provided by most video cameras are generally not equal to the high-resolution images produced by today's better digital cameras. If you need still images in addition to video, you may want to take both types of cameras with you when you conduct your investigation.

One of the biggest advantages to video cameras as compared to still cameras is that many of today's video systems have a night shot function that will allow you to produce video in conditions where there is little natural light. This can be a tremendous asset to the dive accident investigator.

There will undoubtedly be times when you need both still and full motion video images. For example, if you are investigating a recreational accident that took place on a shipwreck, you will probably need to provide a perspective on the overall wreck, or the path the diver followed during the course of the dive. Video is also invaluable if you are involved with the testing of the dive gear.

© *Light and Motion Industries. All rights reserved.*

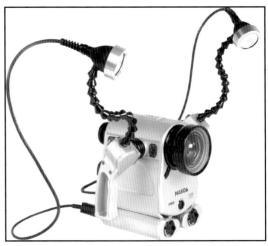

Fig. 6.2 Today's digital video cameras are extremely compact. You can transport an entire underwater video system in a case that will fit under an airline seat. (© Light and Motion Industries. All rights reserved.)

Risk Recognition for Divers and Diving Professionals

Diving is an equipment intensive activity and it's essential that a diver's gear be maintained properly. This means that everyone who is paid to maintain equipment must have the proper factory authorized training, use the original manufacturer's replacement parts, and perform repairs with the proper tools. If you deviate from these parameters, the responsibility for anything that goes wrong with that piece of gear will appropriately rest upon you.

Don't be tempted to work on equipment for which you are not trained, or to use third party spares, or anything other than the required tools. The risks are simply too high for your customers, employees, and yourself.

Be sure to also document any maintenance that you perform, preferably in some type of logbook, so that there is a tangible record that shows when the gear was last serviced and what work was done.

The minimum file size to produce a good 8X10 enlargement from a digital still camera is 3 megapixels. Of course, if you need to make poster size enlargements that are big enough to display in court you will need a file size of roughly 5 megapixels and a wide format printer. Many copy shops can now print poster size enlargements from digital cameras, but your file size needs to be sufficient to get a good print.

Whether or not you use video will be determined by the type of investigation you are conducting, the dive site, and other factors. In most cases, it is better to collect any type of information you think you may need, because it is usually difficult to return to gather information later.

There are excellent underwater housings available now for many digital cameras, so taking a digital camera underwater is not logistically difficult. In addition, since many of these cameras and housings are quite compact, your camera will have excellent protection from rain and boat spray in marine and tropical environments.

You will need some method to transfer the images from your camera to your laptop. Some cameras use special cards that can be read by most laptops, while others can be connected to your computer by a cable. When you purchase these items you'll need to ascertain the capabilities of each device.

With the almost universal availability of software for the digital manipulation of photographs, it is simple for both film and digital photographs to be altered in a computer. There are digital cameras available, specifically designed for legal purposes, that will lock the file so that there can be no charges of digital manipulation.

Digital video with a computer interface allows you to add computer generated graphics to help the viewer better visualize and understand complex visual inter-relationships.

Laptop Computer

In today's world, a laptop computer is an essential tool for the dive accident investigator. The laptop will allow you to be mobile in your investigation, provide a means for you to view your digital photos at large size, and help you to prepare flawless reports. It will also allow you to search for information in electronic databases.

Your laptop should be equipped with a fast modem and/or Ethernet for access to cable modems (or DSL) and to allow you to access a network and share files. The minimum software you will need, aside from your operating system, would include a word processor, photo manipulation software (such as Adobe

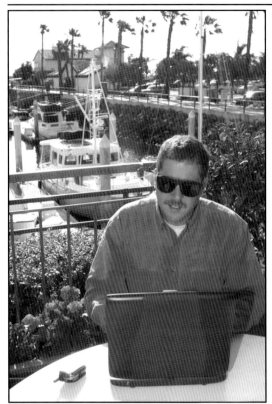

Fig. 6.3 With a laptop computer you can work quite efficiently while you are on the road.

Photoshop®), scanning software (for interfacing with a flatbed scanner) and a page layout program for laying out your report in an organized professional manner. A simple drawing program that will allow you to produce neat sketches of a site or boat is also essential.

Most serious investigators will have access to both a desktop machine as well as a laptop. Although you can open your photos to check the general exposure of the image on a laptop, most laptops only display "thousands of colors," rather than the "millions of colors" that most desktop machines can handle. If color is critical to your photos, you will need a desktop machine as well.

Another important advantage to traveling with a laptop is the ability to work while traveling. If you travel out of town to conduct your investigation, a laptop will allow you to use time on the plane or in a hotel room to your best advantage. In addition, you can keep up with your

email and send reports back to the office with your laptop.

To protect the security of your data, your computer should be protected with a hardware firewall to prevent access by unauthorized persons on the Internet if you are connected to the web via a cable modem or DSL. If you have a wireless connection ("WiFi") then a software firewall should be installed.

Flatbed Scanner

Flatbed scanners are electronic devices that allow you to "copy" flat documents and digitize them. Flatbed scanners will allow you to digitize documents, printed photographs, and photographic negatives.

It is much easier and neater to scan documents into your computer and to add typewritten notes or comments in your report, than to use an office copier and make handwritten notes.

Handheld Organizer

As an adjunct to your computer system, you should consider using a handheld organizer (also known as a "personal digital assistant" or "PDA"). These devices are invaluable in helping you to

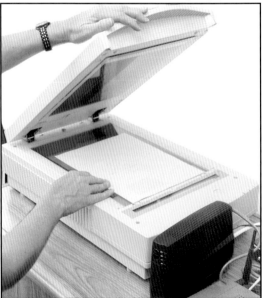

Fig. 6.4 You'll need a scanner to incorporate documents into your report.

schedule appointments and jot down quick notes, especially when carrying a laptop may be inconvenient.

One of the most valuable features of the handheld organizer is its ability to schedule repeating events and alarms to remind you when its time to perform a particular activity. Most handhelds will also interface with your desktop or laptop, allowing you to back-up all of your data including contact information, appointments, billing, etc.

One of the best accessories for many handheld systems today is the addition of a folding keyboard. These devices will allow you to travel with a lightweight system that will still permit you to work on your reports. This may be best if you must fly to a remote location to conduct an investigation and want to carry everything with you aboard the plane.

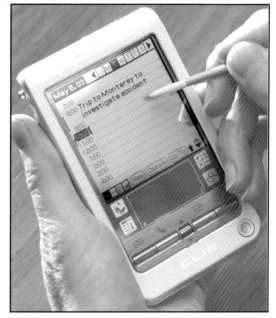

Fig. 6.5 A personal digital assistant is an excellent tool to assist you in planning your investigation.

Color Inkjet or Laser Printer

The range of color inkjet printers today is remarkable, especially when you compare the quality of their output to their low cost. It is possible today for anyone to produce professional reports that combine text, photographs, and charts. A good quality printer is an essential tool to produce these types of documents. The only drawback to most inkjet printers is that they are slow when they are printing in the photo quality mode.

For an inkjet printer to produce a color photograph as part of a page layout program you will need some type of Postscript® interpreter software. These printers rely on your computer to process the data for printing since the inkjet has no "brains" of its own.

If you work full time in the business of producing investigations and need to produce reports quickly, there is no substitute for a color laser printer. These printers combine high quality with exceptional speed. In addition, since most laser printers are Postscript® devices, a problem with their software is less likely.

Voice Recorder

Every investigator has his own style of conducting interviews, and you will need to discover what works best for you. Some investigators prefer to record each interview for reference, while others prefer to rely on notes. It doesn't matter which method you use, so long as you can produce an accurate report.

Most people are somewhat uncomfortable being recorded, so if it's important that the person you are interviewing be relaxed and comfortable, it may be better not to tape-record your interviews.

Some people may decline to be recorded. However, if the person you are interviewing is insured by your client, one of the clauses of their insurance policy may state that they must cooperate with any investigation conducted by the company. In this circumstance, it is best to let the attorney representing the insured explain the consequences of non-cooperation.

If you are interviewing someone for the purposes of an insurance investigation, some attorneys will prefer that you do not record any of your interviews. Conversely, some attorneys insist that every interview should be tape recorded and transcribed. You will need to determine exactly what your client wants if you are doing this type of work.

Dive Gear

In some cases, you will need to dive the site where the accident took place in order to have a full grasp of the realities of the accident. This won't always be the case, but as an investigator you need to be prepared to do this.

You should have good quality dive gear in top condition that is ready to go whenever you are called upon to investigate an accident. It is unprofessional to cause a delay in an investigation because your equipment is in poor repair.

Ideally, your dive computer should be the type that will interface with a desktop or laptop computer so that you can produce a hard copy printout of your dive for your records and report.

Fiberglass Measuring Tape

A fiberglass measuring tape is a frequent tool for the dive accident investigator. It can be used to measure almost anything, from the deck of a dive boat to the position of rocks on a beach. Since you will be taking measurements in the marine environment, a fiberglass tape makes more sense than a traditional metal "tape."

In accidents where a diver has been struck by a boat, a fiberglass tape can be used to take the dimensions and relative positions of the features of the bottom of the boat. You will need to attach some type of clips to the start of the tape so that you can fasten it to the boat if necessary as you make measurements.

Slate

If you need to dive to inspect a site or take measurements on the bottom of a boat, you will need a diver's slate for recording information. The easiest way to handle a slate is to attach it to a spring loaded retractor attached to your buoyancy compensator.

Retractors are spring-loaded reels that unravel when you pull the slate out to use it and automatically reel the slate back in once you release it.

Magnifying Glass

Most of the serial numbers etched into dive equipment are small and can be difficult to read. In addition, some defects in equipment can also be difficult to detect with the naked eye. A good magnifying glass will help you to identify these items correctly.

Chalk

Many pieces of diving equipment are manufactured from black plastic and the serial numbers for these items are frequently molded into this material. Even

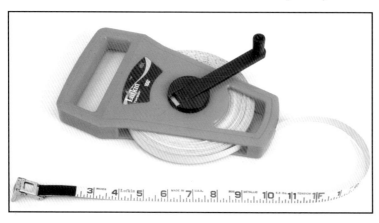

Fig. 6.6 Fiberglass measuring tapes are essential for taking measurements on boats and at dive sites.

using a magnifying glass, it may be difficult to see and correctly identify numbers in this type of situation. Photographs of serial numbers etched into black plastic are almost impossible to read.

Ordinary white chalk can be rubbed across etched numbers and the chalk will stick in the grooves caused by the mold. Brush off the excess chalk and the numbers will be relatively easy to read or photograph.

Handheld GPS

The Global Positioning System (GPS) is a network of satellites that are in orbit around the earth, and are designed to transmit position information to electronic receivers on the surface of the planet. These receivers interpret the distance to each satellite and by calculating the differences between their locations, provide the user of the receiver with his precise location. Most people refer to these units as "GPS receivers" or just simply "GPS."

Since many locations on nautical charts do not have formal names, the use of a GPS receiver will allow you to pinpoint the exact location of an incident and other critical locations that may have played a role in the incident. In addition to providing location information, a GPS unit will provide you with distances between locations. For example, you can "capture" the location information for the dock where the dive boat departed, and once you arrive at the site of interest, you will then be able to calculate the distance between the two. Similarly, most GPS units will track the speed at which you are moving towards a known location, so you could also measure the speed of the dive boat.

Many GPS units will allow you to download both nautical charts and street maps from compact disks loaded into your computer. If your investigations take you out of town to locations with which you are unfamiliar, a GPS unit can be invaluable for finding your way.

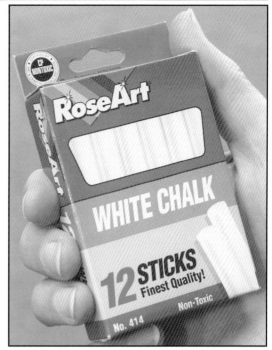

Fig. 6.7 If you rub chalk into the serial numbers etched into most dive gear they will be easier to read.

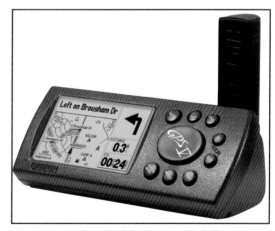

Fig. 6.8 A handheld GPS will help you to find locations you must visit and accurately identify the location of the dive site and its features. (Photo courtesy Garmin Corporation.)

Oxygen Analyzer

If you investigate sport diving accidents where nitrox, tri-mix or a rebreather was involved, or you investigate commercial diving accidents, you'll definitely want your own oxygen analyzer for checking the gas mixture used by the victim. These electronic devices are

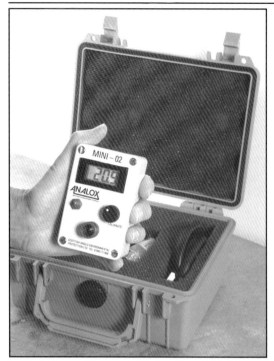

Fig. 6.9 To check the percentage of oxygen in a gas mixture, you'll need an oxygen analyzer.

Air Sample Kit

There are several specialized labs that provide equipment for taking air samples from scuba sources. In most cases, these labs will provide you with a kit that you can use to take an air sample from a high or low-pressure compressor, or a high-pressure gas cylinder. The kit is then returned to the lab where the air is analyzed and a report or certificate is sent back to you. It's not necessary for you to buy the air sample kit itself. You pay only for the analysis.

If you have never taken an air sample before, be sure to read the instructions that are provided with the kit carefully before you go into the field to take the test. If there is something in the instructions you don't understand, call the supplier of the kit and ask them to explain it to you. Don't wait until you are on site to try to figure out how to use the apparatus.

easy to operate and give a precise reading of the mixture in the cylinder being checked. They can be readily calibrated using room air.

Other Specialized Equipment

Depending on the type of investigation you are conducting, you may find you need other specialized equipment.

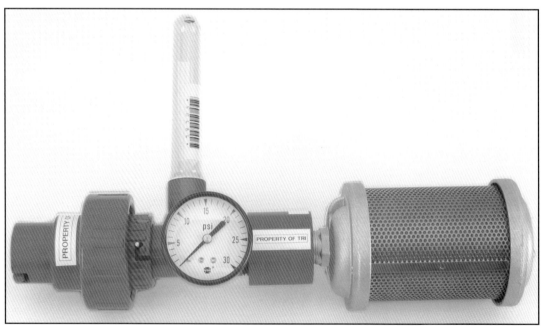

Fig. 6.10 To properly analyze the diver's breathing air, you'll need to take a sample with a test kit like this one. (Equipment courtesy of Texas Research Institute)

For example, if you are investigating an accident involving a semi-closed circuit rebreather, you may need a highly accurate flow meter to check the gas flow through the system.

Charts and Maps

For any investigation you will need nautical charts and street maps of points of interest related to the incident. The nautical charts will help you verify the depth and exact location of the incident. Even if you have a mapping GPS you will need the ability to print and/or include charts in your report.

Street maps are important for your report if the incident took place during a shore dive to show information such as access points, hospitals, police stations, fire stations, and other similar information. The maps will also allow you to calculate relative distances so that you can put victim transport times or emergency response times into perspective. Additional maps as a back-up to your GPS will allow "the big picture" to become apparent to the recipients of your report.

Case History – Recreational Rebreather Diving

A resort dive operation offered training in the use of a semi-closed circuit nitrox rebreather. The training was extensive and was conducted under the auspices of a nationally recognized diver training agency.

An instructor for the resort was conducting one of the rebreather courses with a group of three students. During the first openwater dive, everything seemed to be going smoothly. Upon completing the required exercises, the instructor was leading the students on an underwater tour of the dive site when one of the students lagged behind and disappeared. Fortunately, the instructor noticed that the student was missing almost immediately, and located the student who was revived.

When the police arrived at the scene and recovered the diving equipment, they confiscated the gear and placed it in an evidence locker. It was stored as it was retrieved, assembled and still dripping with salt water. No attempt was made to clean or break down the gear.

Following the incident, the student was hospitalized for 24 hours for observation and released. Shortly thereafter, the individual retained a lawyer and filed a lawsuit.

During the course of the investigation, it was revealed to the investigator that the rebreather had not been properly checked to ensure that it was operational prior to the dive. One of the checks with this type of rebreather is a flow check to confirm the correct amount of breathing gas is being delivered to the diver.

The diving equipment was picked up at the police department by the plaintiff's attorney and the defense investigator. When the rebreather was tested, it was determined that the rebreather did not provide the correct amount of gas during the specified time period. Whether the rebreather was functioning properly during the dive, or whether corrosion occurred due to a lack of maintenance following the dive which then lead to a failure of the flow test, could not be determined. The plaintiff's attorney maintained that the gear was not functioning properly during the dive, while the defense maintained that the rebreather's poor performance was due to improper storage. Had an investigator been dispatched immediately, it is possible an independent facility could have examined the equipment and resolved the issue.

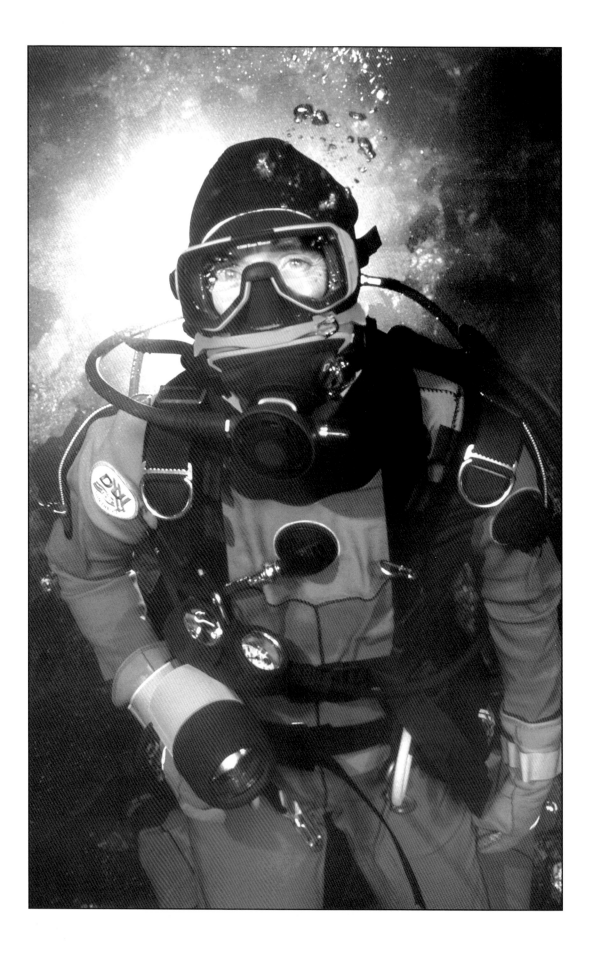

Chapter 7
Preparing for an Investigation

Prior to starting an investigation, your first step is to read and review any documents you may already have concerning the incident. Carefully scan the documents for any facts that will help you formulate your plan. Start to develop your chronology, identify key witnesses, determine where the gear is being held, and locate the site on a map or nautical chart.

Before you set foot in the field, you should know what questions you intend to ask, who you must contact and where, and schedule any possible interviews you may want to conduct.

If you go into the field unprepared, you will undoubtedly need to either return to the site or make numerous follow-up calls after you've returned to the office.

Unless you know all of the people involved in the accident and are intimately familiar with the dive site, it's almost always essential to visit the site and conduct your interviews in person. It is extremely difficult to conduct an effective investigation over the telephone and many people will not discuss these matters unless they can meet you in person.

It is often difficult to secure documents from public agencies without a personal visit. In many cases, you can obtain documents that might not normally be made available if you establish a relationship with the people in charge.

You'll need to have any required re-

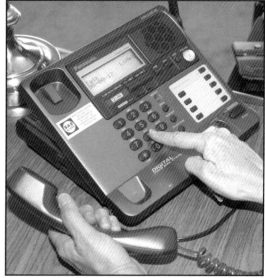

Fig. 7.1 Be sure to schedule all of your interviews ahead of time to ensure that the people you need to speak with are available.

leases with you as you attempt to collect documentary evidence. In most jurisdictions, Medical Examiner's reports are a matter of public record, but if an autopsy has been performed at a hospital it may become part of the medical record and require a release, or a subpoena.

Selecting People to Interview

One of the most critical aspects in preparing for your investigation is deciding who to interview and in what order. In most cases, it will be fairly obvious whom you should talk to, although your schedule will usually be determined by an individual's availability rather than your convenience or preferences.

The list of people who you should interview will be largely determined by the type of accident and where it took place. The list is slightly different for commercial and professional diving accidents compared to recreational accidents.

If you are investigating a fatality, it is important to try to interview both the coroner's investigator and the Medical Examiner to determine their knowledge of the circumstances. Furthermore, it is extremely useful to determine the reasoning the Medical Examiner used to make his diagnosis. There have been circumstances where a diagnosis of drowning was made merely because the victim had wrinkled toes.

Selecting People to Interview in Recreational Diving Accidents

In a recreational diving accident, you will generally want to interview the following people:

- Any instructor who was on site – instructors usually understand their observations better than the average diver.
- Any divemaster who was on site
- Any assistant instructor who was on site
- The victim's buddy
- Other divers who were present at the site
- Any rescuers who responded to the incident
- The dive store owner (if the incident took place during a store organized dive or instruction) or if gear was rented from a store
- Any personnel from the store who dealt with the victim
- The boat captain
- Deckhands on the boat
- Any other bystanders who may have witnessed any portion of the incident
- You should at least make an attempt

to talk to medical personnel, chamber operators, and EMS providers, although in most cases, these individuals will not speak with you

If the rescuers were leadership level divers from another training agency other than that of the insured instructor or divemaster, and you are conducting an investigation for an attorney who has been retained by an insurance company, you should obtain permission from the agency to which the rescuers belong before attempting to interview their members. In most cases, you will **not** get permission to interview the members of another training agency from the agency or its attorneys.

Selecting People to Interview in Professional Diving Accidents

Since professional diving operations may be conducted on scuba or with surface-supplied breathing gas, the list of people to interview may be more like the list for recreational incidents or commercial incidents, depending on the mode of diving. In some situations in professional diving, there may be no diving supervisor on site, (i.e., when two scientists go out to collect specimens, the dive team will normally consist of only these divers).

Selecting People to Interview in Commercial Diving Accidents

In a commercial diving accident, you will usually interview the following people:
- The diving supervisor
- The tender
- The standby diver
- The rack operator (manifold operator)
- Other tenders on deck
- Other divers on deck
- The vessel captain (barge supervisor or installation manager)

- The deckhands on the vessel
- Company management

If you can conduct your interview at the job site, it will be much easier for the people who were involved to explain things and demonstrate where things took place.

Developing Interview Questions

Out of necessity, interview questions will be based upon the information available at the start of the investigation. As your inquiries proceed, the scope and focus of your questions may change. At a minimum, your questions should cover all of the basic lines of inquiry, including "who, what, where, why, when, and how" types of questions.

Your questions for the people involved will combine both open-ended questions and close-ended questions. Open-ended questions deal with concepts, interpretations of events, and descriptions of behaviors. Open-ended questions might include the following:

- When you first arrived on the scene, what was the instructor doing?
- How was the victim brought to the surface?

Closed-ended questions refer to questions that can be answered only with facts, often with one word answers. Closed-ended questions leave little room for opinions or additional information. Examples of good closed-ended questions might include:

- What time did the Coast Guard arrive on site?
- Who called the sheriff's department?
- What was the distance from the victim to the boat?

Develop a Plan for Gear Inspection

If you know that you will be inspecting diving equipment, be sure to develop a written plan for the items that you want to examine. This is helpful for several reasons. First, if you will be inspecting new gear that is not familiar to you, you need to anticipate any special equipment you might need for your inspection. For example, if you need to flow check a semi-closed circuit rebreather, like a Drager, you will want to be sure to have a flow meter available for performing your test. Or, if you need to check the percentage of oxygen in a gas mixture, you will need an oxygen analyzer.

By having a written plan, you will also be sure that you do not forget to check any items. This will also allow you to go back and confirm what you did if there is ever a question in the future.

Locating Resources

There are a number of ways to gather information that will help you identify resources. If the dive was conducted from a boat, you should be able to get a copy of the manifest from the captain of the boat. If a Coast Guard or police report already exists, this may also identify key participants in the incident.

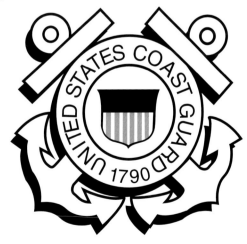

Fig. 7.2 The Coast Guard will almost always have a report on any fatality that took place at sea.

Large land-based resorts will often have their own security personnel who usually respond to any incident on their property and file their own internal report. These documents may be made readily available to you if you approach their personnel with a good attitude. Although you may not be allowed to photocopy the extensive report in a hotel's file, with the proper approach you may be allowed to read the report and make extensive notes on its contents.

The Internet, Newspapers, and Libraries

Prior to your trip into the field, spend some time on the Internet looking for information on the victim. One of your first stops should be the large search engines on the Internet. Type in the person's name and city and see if anything comes up. Be careful if the person has a common name, such as Joe Smith, to be sure that any articles that you retrieve are referring to the right Joe Smith. If you have a telephone number, enter that information. You may then be able to find out the location of the phone. There are also a variety of Internet sites that provide aerial pictures of specific addresses.

If you don't get any results from the search engines, next check to see if the hometown newspaper of the victim has a website. If the paper is on-line, check to see if they maintain archives of back issues. If so, check through these archives to locate any articles about the victim.

If there are no archives on-line, get the phone number of the paper and give them a call to determine how long they maintain back issues of the paper for sale and how to obtain them. You will want copies of the paper for at least a week following the incident.

If your investigation takes place beyond the date at which the newspaper maintains back issues for sale, you will need to visit the local library to scan back issues for any relevant articles. Most

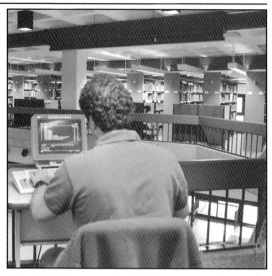

Fig. 7.3 Preparation before you go into the field is key. This preparation may include Internet research, library research, or visits to the local newspaper.

libraries keep hard copies of the local paper for the last two or three months, before sending them out to be transferred to microfilm or microfiche. Check out the location of the library, their hours, and whether they maintain copies of the paper and what provisions they may have for copying microfilm or microfiche.

Request Long Lead Documents Immediately

Certain documents may take a long time to obtain and you should request these items as soon as you have been assigned an investigation. For example, in Los Angeles County, it frequently takes months to obtain an autopsy report, due to the huge volume of autopsies the coroner's office must process, and the large number of requests they get for these documents. In some jurisdictions you can go to the office of the medical examiner and look at the autopsy with minimal lead time.

Similarly, it may take a long time to obtain U.S. Coast Guard logs once you have filed a "FOIA" (Freedom of Information Act) request for this information.

Make your request, in writing, to the Coast Guard office you suspect handled the incident as soon as you have been assigned a particular investigation.

Check with Every Local Agency

It's important to check with every local agency that may have responded to the incident to be sure that you have not overlooked any information. For example, in the United States, the local fire department will generally respond to almost any incident that requires life-saving measures be administered.

Fire departments will readily share any information they consider "public," such as their response log times. Information on any medical procedures will not be released to private individuals and will need to be subpoenaed if they are required in a legal case.

Coroner's reports will not be available to an insurance investigator in certain jurisdictions without a court order. This can vary from county to county, even in the same state. In the event the case has not been cleared by the police department and is still under investigation as a possible homicide, the coroner's report will be unavailable until the case has cleared. Again, if you are investigating on behalf of an insurance company, or as an expert witness, you will usually be most successful if you visit the agency from which you are soliciting information, personally. Most public service agency personnel tend to distrust people who they have never met in person.

Scheduling Interviews

If you must interview private individuals, you will want to make it as convenient as possible for these people to cooperate with you. In most cases this will mean that your interviews will be conducted in the evenings, at lunchtime, or on weekends. Work around people's schedules; don't expect them to conform to yours.

The advantages of scheduling interviews are that you can usually count on most people making themselves available to you, and you can make the most efficient use of your time. The disadvantage of scheduling interviews is that it gives people time to think about and "plan" their responses, to the extent that they can anticipate what your questions might be.

Call the people you want to interview well in advance of your visit to be sure that they will be available when you want to meet with them. This is particularly important if your investigation is taking place out of town. Ideally, you'll want to

Risk Recognition for Divers and Diving Professionals

In any sport diving operation involving a group of divers in training or on a trip, it's vital that there be a clear chain of command in the event an accident occurs. It's also essential to have a plan of action so that everyone who is in a position of responsibility knows what is expected of them and how they should respond.

In most sport diving operations, the person in charge will usually be a diving instructor, who will be assisted by either assistant instructors or divemasters. While this chain of command is usually well recognized, few dive operators take the time to rehearse how they will handle an incident when it occurs. Even though all leadership personnel will have rescue training, there's no substitute for practicing as a team with the people who you work with at the actual dive site you use for training. A drill should be conducted so that each individual has the opportunity to fulfill various roles and a debrief should follow each run through of the procedures. This will provide the best possible care for your divers.

interview them in a location where they feel comfortable meeting you.

If you want any documents from the individuals you will be interviewing, be sure to ask for them to be ready when you arrive. You don't want to arrive on site and find out there is no copy machine or to waste time making copies when you could be using your time productively.

In a sport diving accident, be sure to obtain copies of the following:

- All training records relating to the victim
- All receipts for diving services and equipment purchased by the victim
- All rental records for equipment used by the victim on the day of the accident
- All maintenance records for rental equipment used by the victim on the day of the accident
- Air compressor sample records
- Air compressor maintenance records
- Vessel logs
- Copies of the download from the victim's dive computer
- Copies of the download from the instructor's dive computer (if the accident happened during instruction)
- Any waivers or releases
- The victim's dive log
- The buddy's dive log
- A download of the buddy's dive computer
- Download and logs for other people who may have been on the dive if neither the victim or his partner's logs are available

In a commercial diving accident, aside from public agency documents, you'll want to collect copies of the following documents:

- The dive log for the accident
- The job log
- The gas analyzation for any mixed gas dive
- Records of mixed gas purchases
- Air sample reports from the compressor
- Equipment maintenance records for all gear used on the job
- Vessel logs
- Copies of the victim's personal dive logbook
- Copies of the victim's personnel records
- Any variances the company has obtained for conducting their operations outside normal regulations

These documents will need to be compared to government regulations and industry standards.

Check Out Your Equipment

If there is any special equipment that you will need for your investigation, be sure to check it out and ensure that it is working a few days in advance of the time you will need it. Test your micro-cassette recorder, video camera, or diving gear if you haven't used them in some time.

If you need film, batteries, or micro-cassette tapes, be sure to have these on hand, all well as replacements, as they may be difficult to locate if you are traveling out of town, or especially out of the country.

Know Where Everything is Located

If you are traveling out of town, take some time before you leave to know where each person or agency you must visit is located and how to get there relative to your hotel. This will allow you to plan your time so you are most productive.

The best resource for planning is the Internet. There are numerous map sites that will not only provide you with maps but also driving directions. A GPS unit that has road maps and voice directions in it can be a real time saver, especially if you must frequently travel to cities that are unfamiliar to you.

Case History – Recreational Divers

A group of three divers decided to dive along a rugged stretch of the west coast of the U.S. One of them owned an inflatable which they launched off the beach in a protected cove. Two of the divers were very experienced, but the third was not.

They motored the boat down the coast to a rocky reef where the two more experienced divers had been diving on a previous trip. After entering the water, they set out to explore the reef at a depth of 80 FSW.

Midway through the dive, the less experienced diver became separated from the other two, who were unable to locate their friend. They searched until they ran out of air, then ascended and returned to the cove where they had launched their boat and called for help.

Sheriff's divers arrived within the hour, but were unable to locate the missing diver. By late afternoon, sea conditions had become rough and the search had to be abandoned. Although the sheriff's deputies returned to the site several times to look for the missing diver, the search was ultimately abandoned.

Several weeks later, divers from the missing diver's home town returned to the dive site to attempt to locate the body. On the second dive of the day, they found the missing diver, who they successfully brought to the surface, but were unable to pull into the boat. Rather than remove the dead diver's gear or call for help, they tied a rope around his tank and towed the body back to the beach.

At some point during the tow, the diver's weight belt became loose and was lost. When they reached the cove, the body was towed over rocks and across the pebbled bottom. The coroner and the sheriff's department came to pick up the body shortly after the dive team arrived back at the beach.

The family of the diver filed suit against the store that had rented him the equipment, claiming that the gear was defective. Although some of the gear was obviously damaged, there was no way to know for sure its exact condition when it was rented, or whether the damage had occurred when the body was towed back to the beach across the rocks.

When the investigator for the insurance company finally had the opportunity to inspect the equipment, it had been stored unrinsed, in a hot aircraft hanger, where aviation fuel was leaking. There was no way to determine how long the equipment had been stored in that environment, or what damage had taken place due to the heat or fumes from the fuel.

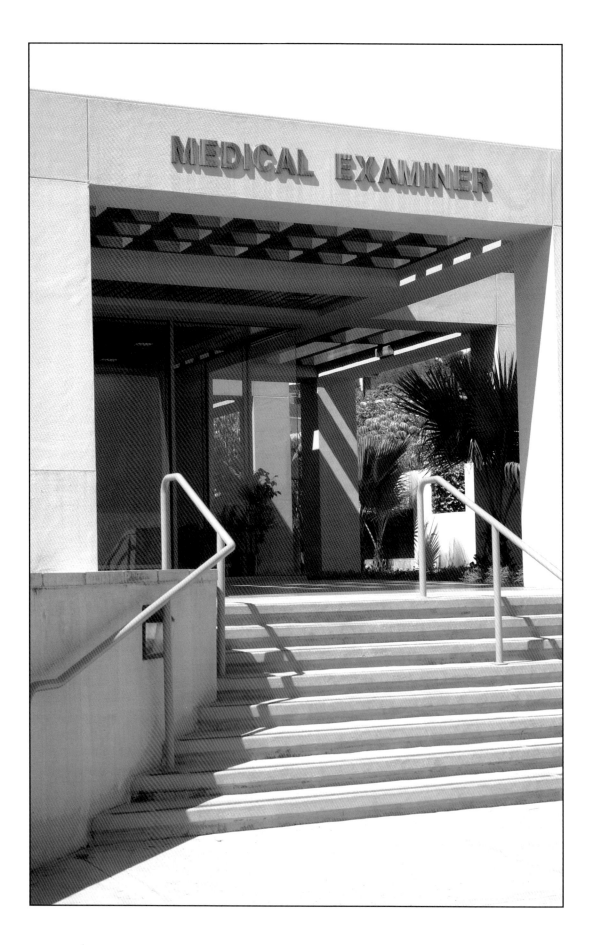

Chapter 8
Conducting an Investigation

As already mentioned in the introduction to this book, most victims of both fatal and non-fatal diving accidents are recovered by other divers who happen to be on the site when the accident takes place. This is true in both recreational diving accidents and commercial diving accidents.

Since recreational diving tends to be a social activity, that takes place in the company of other people, there are almost always other divers around when an accident occurs. Likewise, commercial diving activities are conducted by teams of divers working together, and in a responsible operation, there is typically a standby diver prepared to go to the aid of an incapacitated diver.

All divers recognize the need for the rapid rescue and recovery of a person who has become unconscious underwater. It is rare for a missing diver to be left underwater with no immediate attempt made to recover the victim, and in most cases, recovery is successful. This makes a true underwater forensic investigation rare, and forces the dive accident investigator to rely on accounts of the incident provided by other people.

Conducting personal interviews is the most difficult aspect of investigating diving accidents. Not only must you know the right questions to ask, but you also must be sensitive to the reactions of the person whom you are questioning. Whenever you interview a person from the general public who has been directly involved with a diving accident, you must be prepared to deal with someone who is emotionally upset, frightened, and possibly hostile towards you.

Many people experience some degree of survivor guilt following a diving accident and almost all experience sadness and a sense of loss. Your attitude and demeanor during your interview can make or break the success of your investigation.

It's essential to remember to avoid forming any opinions or formulating any theories about what took place until you have completed your investigation. Different people observe the same event from different perspectives (both physical and mental) and may make very different observations and reach radically different conclusions about what occurred.

In a sport diving situation, novice divers in particular may make incorrect observations or not understand what they have seen, and their reports should always be viewed with a certain amount of skepticism. In a commercial diving situation, apprentice divers (tenders) may not fully comprehend what took place during an accident.

Your Personal Appearance is Important

Like it or not, people do judge you based on your appearance, so you want to be sure that you project the right image

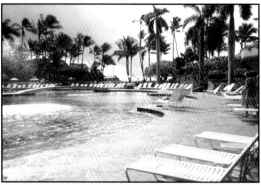

Fig. 8.1 At a tropical resort, it's usually appropriate if you are dressed in conservative shorts and a polo shirt while conducting your investigation.

when you conduct investigations. While this doesn't mean that you necessarily need to wear a business suit, you do need to have a professional appearance and dress appropriately.

If you are going to be conducting interviews in a dive store or people's homes in the mainland U.S., you'll want to wear a nice pair of slacks and a clean, collared shirt. Blue jeans, cut-off shorts, T-shirts, and tank tops are not advised. Obviously, if you are visiting a police department, fire department, or other public agency, you want to be appropriately attired.

Conversely, if you are conducting an investigation in a location like Hawaii, where the weather is warm, you can wear a polo shirt, conservative shorts, and boat shoes and be considered appropriately dressed. Similarly, if your investigation takes you to a dive site or out aboard a dive boat, you'll want to dress appropriately, without being over-dressed or under-dressed. Your goal is to fit in without drawing attention to yourself.

Avoid Criticism or Suggestions

Probably the most important thing that you can do when you conduct an interview following a diving accident is to studiously avoid being judgmental in your reaction to how the event was handled. This is equally important whether you are interviewing rescuers, instruc-

tional personnel, the victim, his buddy, or other divers.

If you are a diving instructor, it can be especially difficult to conceal your feelings about any mistakes you feel were made by the instructor managing the accident. However, it is critical to avoid expressing your personal opinions.

Don't Cue Your Witness

As you near the end of your interviews, when you think you have a good idea about what happened, it's easy to begin to form opinions about what took place. This is the time when you must maintain an open mind so that you remain receptive to new information that may change your view about what transpired.

It's also essential to avoid cueing your witnesses, not just as your interviews draw to a close, but at any time. Things may not have taken place quite like you think and if you supply too much information to those you are interviewing you may bias the way in which they report their information to you.

Interview One Person at a Time

Always try to avoid interviewing more than one person at a time. This is especially important whenever you have a situation where one person may be the more highly experienced diver, such as a father and son dive team. There is a natural tendency for the less experienced diver to defer in their opinions and observations to the more experienced diver and change their viewpoint as a result. Always try to interview each diver individually, unless you have no other choice.

Be Prepared to Change Your Questions

Even though you should always go to an interview with a prepared list of questions, in almost all cases witnesses or those involved will give you new information that will require you to develop additional questions. Be sure to note down any additional questions as you think of them so that you don't forget them.

Audio Recording of Interviews

Even if you tape or digitally record the interview, it's still a good idea to take notes just in case the recorder fails. It's also a good idea in case any portions of the tape are unintelligible due to background noise or other problems. Always be sure to take spare batteries or an AC adapter with you as well as more than sufficient recording media to cover all of the interviews with media to spare.

Some attorneys (clients) want every interview tape recorded or video taped, while others do not. You will need to determine the preferences of each attorney with whom you work.

Some people will not want to be tape recorded. Of course, if you are not a police investigator conducting an investigation you must ask permission before you tape record anyone. The first question on your tape should always be made in regards to securing the permission of the person being interviewed to be recorded.

If you tape record the interview, you will still need to have the tapes transcribed for your report. The transcriber must be a person who you can trust to be discreet and hold the information in confidence. Always start the recording by identifying yourself, the date, the location, and the person being interviewed, as well as the case.

At the completion of the interview, lock the tape so that you do not accidentally reuse it and label it with the name of the person interviewed and the date. If you need more than one tape to record the same person, number the tapes sequentially.

After the tapes are transcribed, you will still need to edit the written version because there will often be mistakes in the

transcription. This will occur particularly with a transcriber who is not familiar with diving terms and misunderstands some of the words and phrases.

Videotaping Interviews

Sometimes, it may be advantageous to video the interview, particularly if the person's information may be needed for court and they will be unavailable at a later date. Video conveys more information than audio tapes do.

If you are responsible for recording a video, be sure to set the camera to record the date and time. Use a tripod to provide stability for the recording.

Some people are extremely self-conscious about appearing on camera. Using a tripod will relax many of these people, since you are not looking at them through the viewfinder. Their attention will be drawn to you and not the camera, particularly if the camera is off to the side.

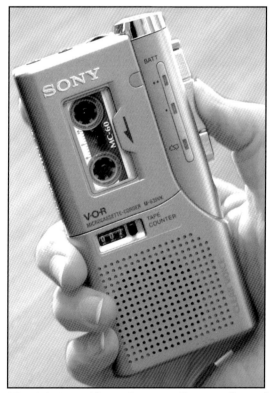

Fig. 8.2 Even if you do an audio recording of the interview, it's still wise to take notes in case the recorder fails.

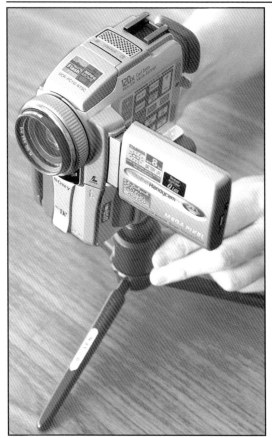

Fig. 8.3 Use a small tripod with your video camera and set the camera slightly off to the side.

Follow the same procedures that you would with an audio tape when your interview is complete. Lock the tape and label it with the name of the person interviewed and the date.

Since the sound portion of a videotape is not usually transcribed, you'll want to make a duplicate copy of the original and store it in a secure location, remote from the original. Both video and audiotapes should be stored vertically (on edge) and not laid flat.

Photographing People

Some attorneys will request that an investigator submit a transcribed audio interview and a still photograph of the person. They want to be able to put a name with a face. Even if your client doesn't ask for photographs, the people who must read your report usually appreciate them.

Most people tense up when you take their photograph. Try to get them to relax so that their photo doesn't end up looking like a mug shot.

Conducting Interviews by Telephone

While it is always better to conduct your interviews in person, there will be times when it is impractical to meet your witness face to face. In these situations, your only choice may be to conduct your interview on the phone. An alternative to the telephone is a teleconference if appropriate facilities are available.

Set up a telephone interview in advance if you can, but be prepared for the fact that some people may want to do the interview the first time you call them. If they are willing to do the interview immediately, you should definitely proceed with your questions, because sometimes people change their minds once they have had time to think about the purpose of your call.

If you plan to record an interview that takes place on the phone, you must inform the person before you start to be sure that they consent to being recorded. If they say they are uncomfortable being recorded, you have no choice but to leave the recorder off.

Visiting a Dive Store Involved in a Sport Diving Accident

If you are investigating a sport diving accident that happened during instruction, you definitely need to visit the store that sponsored the course. In most cases, the store will have a classroom available that you can use to conduct your interviews.

Take a good look around the store so you get a feel for their operation. Before you arrive request copies of any documents you think you'll want for your report.

At the store, take photos of the rental

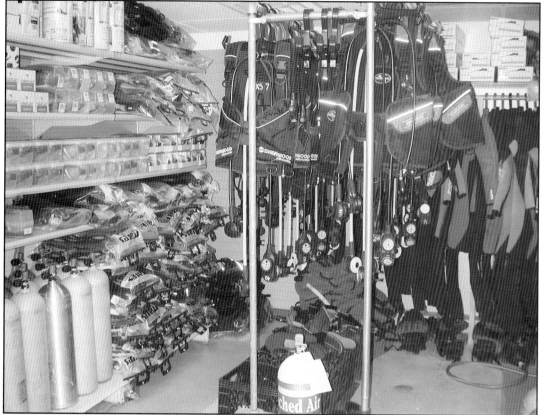

Fig. 8.4 Check out the rental area and repair room of any store you visit for an investigation and photograph them.

area, the repair department, the compressor installation, and any other features you think may be relevant. Note the quality of the records maintained by the store and how they are maintained (by hand, on a computer, on index cards, etc.).

Collect copies of any relevant documents that pertain in any way to the incident. These documents may include:

- Sales receipts for any items purchased by the victim
- Copies of warranty cards for dive gear purchased by the victim
- Newsletters or photographs of the victim taken by the store (even if the photographs were taken at an earlier date)
- Any correspondence between the victim and the store owner (thank-you notes, letters of complaint, etc.)
- Rosters for trips in which the victim participated

- Air sample results
- Waivers and releases

If the accident occurred during an instructional course, you will need to obtain copies of everything in the student's folder. At a minimum this should include the following documents:

- Course application
- Attendance record
- Medical statement
- Copies of quizzes and exams
- Waiver and release

Do not take possession of the original documents unless you have been specifically instructed to do so by the attorney. Advise the storeowner or manager that they should secure all of the original documents pertaining to the case in a safe deposit box or other secure location.

Visiting a Resort or Dive Boat Involved in a Sport Diving Accident

Land based dive resorts are sometimes part of a larger operation, such as an international hotel chain, or the entire resort may be dedicated to diving and/or other watersports. In a land-based resort you may find it more difficult to conduct your investigation, especially if the diving operation is based in a large hotel. This is generally due to the fact that the victim may have spent more of his time engaged in activities other than diving.

Another asset that you may be able to obtain from a land-based resort is a site-map of the property. This type of document can be invaluable to understand what took place and create your report. Also, be sure to pick up copies of any promotional literature used by the resort or boat. This may provide additional information that may be important.

For most vessels larger than a six-passenger dive boat, there will almost always be a log of the vessel's operation. Unfortunately, all too frequently ship's logs on dive boats are not well maintained. Regardless, you should attempt to obtain a copy of the log as it should contain the time the vessel left port, when it arrived on site, and when diving operations commenced. With any luck it will also contain some information regarding the accident, although usually the details on such incidents will not be well documented by the vessel's captain.

All dive boats normally use a check in/check out roster of some type. Each diver's time entering and exiting the water is recorded. This record is used to ensure that everyone is aboard the boat before the boat departs for its next location. In some cases, the roster may be kept on paper so it may be possible to obtain a copy. However, on many boats, the list

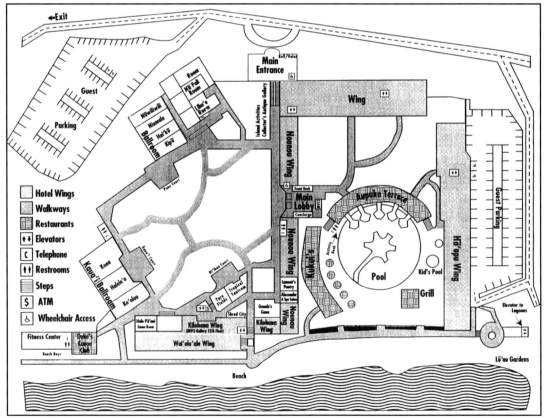

Fig. 8.5 Whenever possible, be sure to obtain a site-map of any land based resort where you are conducting an investigation.

Risk Recognition for Divers and Diving Professionals

Compressors are essential to all types of diving, with the exception of free diving activities and snorkeling. Most diving operations recognize the importance of regular compressor maintenance and the implications of a compressor failure. However, not all companies are as conscientious as they should be about performing regular air quality checks.

Air sampling should be conducted at least once a quarter. Since an air compressor can operate properly one day and deliver "bad" air the next there is never a 100% guarantee that a given system is operating reliably following the results of an air sample. In some cases, divers will report bad air before it gets serious enough to cause an accident, because the air may smell or taste "bad."

Always be extremely responsive in regards to complaints from divers about the quality of air pumped by your compressor. The price of an additional air sample is a small price to help ensure the safety of your divers.

is maintained on a Plexiglas board that is erased at the end of each day, so there may not be a record of the dive times available.

All charter dive boats in the U.S. use a waiver and release of liability that they require all passengers to sign before the trip departs from the dock. Unless you are investigating on behalf of the dive boat itself, you probably will not be able to obtain a copy of this release.

If the victim was participating in a dive trip organized by a dive store or instructor, these entities will generally use their own waiver and release, in addition to the one used by the boat. To be considered effective, the store's (or instructor's) release should be signed by the participants of the trip prior to their arrival at the boat or resort. Be sure to obtain a copy of this document from the trip organizers if you are investigating on their behalf.

Visiting Local Agencies

Probably the most important thing that you can do when visiting any local agency is to establish rapport with the people you meet. Demonstrate by your behavior that you are their colleague, not their enemy. Don't walk in and demand anything. Always ask politely.

If you know people in common that the people at the agency might also know,

don't be afraid to mention their names. If you are active in some aspect of the community that they deal with regularly, make this known. You need to establish trust and credibility if you want cooperation from people.

It's almost always better to attempt to obtain documents in person, rather than over the telephone. There is an immediacy to your presence to which most people will respond in a way which they will not respond over the phone. In addition, people tend to trust people that they can deal with in person more than they will an anonymous voice on the telephone.

Be Prepared to Show I.D.

When you are visiting a local agency, always be prepared to show your identification, if requested. While some documents are available to the general public, many documents are considered confidential and may not be available upon request.

Have Documentation

Be sure to be prepared with whatever documentation you may think you need to obtain the reports that are required for your report. In some jurisdictions, you may need a subpoena to get an autopsy report or a police report. In some cases, a letter from an attorney or insurance company indicating that you are representing them may be sufficient to release other information.

Be Prepared to Pay for Reports and Documents

In most situations, you will be required to pay for copies of any documents that you may request. Although the U.S. Coast Guard does not generally require payment for copies of their logs, most coroners, fire departments, and other agencies will expect to be paid for their reports. In many cases, the fees are in excess of what you would pay for simple photocopying. For example, in Los Angeles County, the fee for even the most basic autopsy usually exceeds $50.00.

Unless the case is a suspected or known homicide, the autopsy will usually not be available until quite some time after the incident occurs. In a large city, like Los Angeles, it can sometimes take as much as a year before a final autopsy report is released. In a situation where you expect it will take some time before the autopsy becomes available, you'll want to program a monthly reminder into your computer calendar to remind yourself to check with the coroner's office to see if the autopsy has been completed.

Visiting the Fire Department

In any diving accident that occurs on the beach or near shore, the local fire department's paramedics will almost always respond. The response log will show you what time they received the call, what time they "rolled out," what time they arrived on site, and what time the patient was loaded into the ambulance. Sometimes you may be able to obtain these logs from the local fire station, but in most cases you will need to go to the fire department's headquarters.

If possible, you may want to also visit the local fire station that responded to the call. In some cases, you may be able to interview the individual firefighters who responded to the incident. If you do interview the firemen, it's important to make it clear to them who you are representing. Don't attempt to interview firemen/paramedics if you know or even suspect that there will be legal action taken against them.

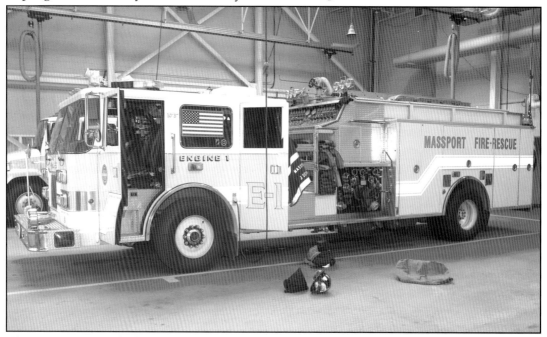

Fig. 8.6 A visit to the fire station that responded to a beach oriented diving accident is almost always productive.

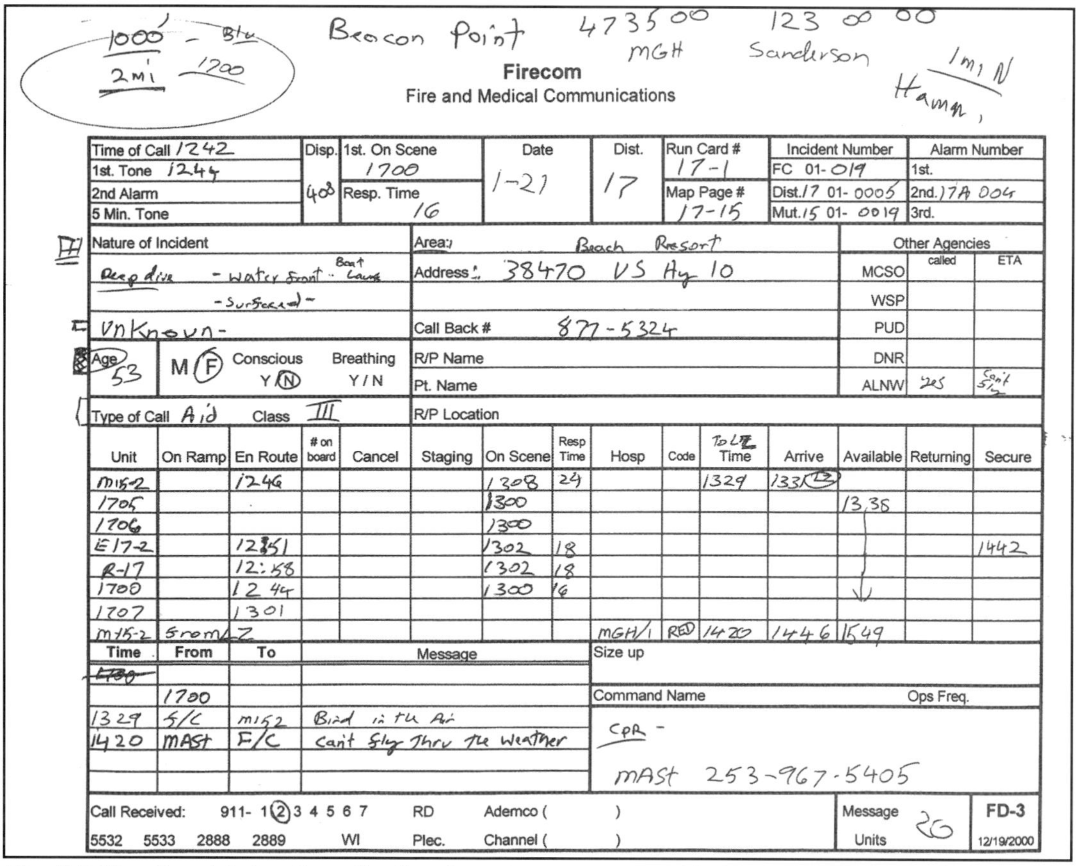

Handwritten notes at top: 1000 - Btu, 2mi - 1200, Beacon Point 473500 mGH 123 00 00 Sanderson 1mi N, Hamn

Firecom
Fire and Medical Communications

Time of Call *1242*	Disp.	1st. On Scene	Date	Dist.	Run Card #	Incident Number	Alarm Number
1st. Tone *1244*		*1700*			*17-1*	FC 01- *019*	1st.
2nd Alarm	*408*	Resp. Time	*1-27*	*17*	Map Page #	Dist.*17* 01- *0005*	2nd.)*7A 004*
5 Min. Tone		*16*			*17-15*	Mut.*15* 01- *0019*	3rd.

Nature of Incident	Area:	Beach Resort	Other Agencies	called	ETA
Deep dive - Water Front Boat Launch - Surfaced -	Address: *38470 US Hy 10*		MCSO		
			WSP		
Unknown -	Call Back # *877-5324*		PUD		
Age *53* M (F) Conscious Y (N) Breathing Y / N	R/P Name		DNR		
	Pt. Name		ALNW	*yes*	*Snk 512*
Type of Call *Aid* Class *III*	R/P Location				

Unit	On Ramp	En Route	# on board	Cancel	Staging	On Scene	Resp Time	Hosp	Code	To LE Time	Arrive	Available	Returning	Secure
M15-2		1246				1308	24			1329	133(13)			
1705						1300						1335		
1706						1300								
E17-2		12:51				1302	18							1442
R-17		12:58				1302	18							
1700		1244				1300	16							
1707		1301												
M15-2	5 rom AZ							mGH/1	RED	1420	1446	1549		

Time	From	To	Message	Size up
~~1730~~	1700			
1329	5/C	M152	Bird in the Air	CPR -
1420	mASt	F/C	cant fly thru the weather	mASt 253-967-5405

		Command Name	Ops Freq.

Call Received:	911- 1 (2) 3 4 5 6 7	RD	Ademco ( )	Message *26*	**FD-3**
5532 5533 2888 2889		WI	Plec.	Channel ( )	Units	12/19/2000

Fig. 8.7 The dispatch log from the fire department can provide important information.

Visiting the Police Department

In larger cities, the local police department will not usually provide you with copies of their reports unless you have a subpoena. You're generally wasting your time in visiting these agencies unless you are with another law enforcement agency or public service agency. The idea of the private investigator who makes up identities or stories to bluff his way into obtaining information is the stuff of television programs, not reality.

You will find the police much more cooperative in smaller cities. In many cases, the police have opened their files to me, driven me to the accident site, and allowed me to photograph and examine equipment. If this is an area where you expect to return, you will do well to share any information with them about diving in general, as long as the information will not compromise your investigation or client.

Visiting the Harbor Master

If the incident took place close to a harbor, there's a chance that one of the agencies that responded was the local harbor patrol. Although these public safety personnel are law enforcement officers, they generally are more relaxed about sharing information than regular police departments.

Visiting the Lifeguards

Lifeguards can provide excellent, reliable information when it comes to any incident that takes place on or about the water. Many lifeguards are sport divers and have a good understanding of diving. There may be reports or logs from the lifeguard services that provide important information.

In some jurisdictions, such as Los Angeles County, the lifeguards have been reassigned from the County Parks Depart-

COUNTY OF LOS ANGELES   DEPARTMENT O

12

AUTOPSY REPORT

No.   −03824

Page ____2____

CIRCUMSTANCES:

The decedent, a 49-year-old Caucasian male, reportedly ran into problems which rendered him unconscious during a scuba dive on ▮▮▮▮▮ at approximately 0750 hours. He was reportedly diving in the Pacific Ocean off the west end of San Clemente Islands. He was taken to the hyperbaric chamber on Catalina Island where he was officially pronounced dead on ▮▮▮▮▮ at 0937 hours. This

---

UNTY OF LOS ANGELES   DEPARTMENT OF

12

AUTOPSY REPORT

No.   −03824

I performed an autopsy on the body of   ➡

the DEPARTMENT OF CORONER

at _____

Los Angeles, California _____ on **MAY 24, 1995 @ 1130 HOURS**
                                       (Date)   (Time)

From the anatomic findings and pertinent history I ascribe the death to:

(A)   **DROWNING**

DUE TO, OR AS A CONSEQUENCE OF

(B)

DUE TO, OR AS A CONSEQUENCE OF

(C)

DUE TO, OR AS A CONSEQUENCE OF

(D)

OTHER CONDITIONS CONTRIBUTING BUT NOT RELATED TO THE IMMEDIATE CAUSE OF DEATH.

      CORONARY ATHEROSCLEROSIS, METHAMPHETAMINE ABUSE

Anatomical Summary:

    I.   Pulmonary edema and congestion, **moderate.**

   II.   Acute visceral congestion, marked.

 III. Cardiomegaly 435 grams.

  IV.   Coronary artery atherosclerosis, moderately severe with 70 to 80% occlusion of the circumflex coronary artery and only slight occlusion, estimated at 10 to 20% of the left main, left anterior descending and right coronary arteries.

   V.   Right ventricular dilatation of the heart.

  VI.   Multiple old scars.

 VII. See microscopic, toxicology and neuropathology reports.

Fig. 8.8 The bottom line in the autopsy is the cause of death. You should always try to get a copy of the autopsy, but in some cities it may not be possible without a subpoena.

STATE OF WASHINGTON
DEPARTMENT OF HEALTH

OFFICE USE ONLY: 1. DISTRICT; 2. COPIES; 3. HOSPITAL; 4. OCCURRENCE; 5. RESIDENCE; 6. TRACT; 7. OCCUPATION; 21. ACC LOC; 22. QUERIES

TYPE OR PRINT IN PERMANENT BLACK INK

Health

CERTIFICATE OF DEATH

LOCAL FILE NUMBER — [redacted] — STATE FILE NUMBER

DECEDENT

Field	Entry
1. NAME (First, Middle, Last)	[redacted]
2. SEX (M / F)	Male
3. DEATH DATE (Mo, Day, Yr)	November [redacted]
4. AGE LAST BIRTHDAY (Yrs)	21
5. UNDER 1 YEAR (Mos, Days)	
6. UNDER 1 DAY (Hours, Mins)	
7. BIRTHDATE (Mo, Day, Yr)	
8. BIRTHPLACE (City, State or Foreign Country)	SALEM, OR.
9. WAS DECEDENT EVER IN U.S. ARMED FORCES? (Yes / No)	NO
10. COUNTY OF DEATH	Snohomish
11. CITY, TOWN OR LOCATION OF DEATH	[redacted]
12. PLACE OF DEATH—X BOX FOR PLACE THEN GIVE ADDRESS OR INSTITUTION NAME (1 HOME, 2 IN TRANSPORT, 3 EMERG RM/OUT PTN, 4 HOSP, 5 NUR HOME, 6 OTHER PLACE)	X 6 OTHER PLACE — Puget Sound- 30 yrds off boat yard
13. SMOKING IN LAST 15 YEARS? (Yes / No)	NO
14. MARITAL STATUS—Married, Never Married, Widowed, Divorced (Specify)	NEVER MARRIED
15. SURVIVING SPOUSE (If wife, give maiden name)	
16. SOCIAL SECURITY NO	[redacted]
17. DECEDENT'S EDUCATION (Specify only highest grade completed) Elementary/Secondary (0-12) / College (1-4 or 5+)	College: 2
18. USUAL OCCUPATION (Give kind of work done during most of working life. DO NOT USE RETIRED)	STUDENT
19. KIND OF BUSINESS OR INDUSTRY	COLLEGE
20. Was Decedent of Hispanic origin or descent? (Ancestry) (Specify Yes or No. If Yes, specify Cuban, Mexican, Puerto Rican, etc.) (Yes / No) Specify	NO
21. RACE (Specify)	[redacted]
22. RESIDENCE—NUMBER AND STREET	[redacted]
23. CITY/TOWN, OR LOCATION	[redacted]
24. INSIDE CITY LIMITS? (Yes / No)	NO
25A. COUNTY	
25B. LENGTH OF RES IN CO.	[redacted] yrs.
26. STATE	OR
27. ZIP CODE	[redacted]

PARENTS

Field	Entry
28. FATHER'S NAME—FIRST, MIDDLE, LAST	[redacted]
29. MOTHER'S NAME—FIRST, MIDDLE, MAIDEN SURNAME	[redacted]
30. INFORMANT—NAME	[redacted]
31. MAILING ADDRESS (STREET OR RFD NO, CITY OR TOWN, STATE, ZIP)	ARROW CT.

DISPOSITION

Field	Entry
32. BURIAL, CREMATION, REMOVAL, OTHER (Specify)	REM/BURIAL
33. DATE (Mo, Day, Yr)	[redacted]
34. CEMETERY/CREMATORY—NAME	CATHOLIC CEMETERY
35. LOCATION—CITY/TOWN, STATE	
36. FUNERAL DIRECTOR SIGNATURE	X [redacted]
37. NAME OF FACILITY	[redacted]
38. ADDRESS OF FACILITY	SEATTLE, WA.

CERTIFIER

TO BE COMPLETED ONLY BY **CERTIFYING PHYSICIAN**

39. **TO THE BEST OF MY KNOWLEDGE**, DEATH OCCURRED AT THE TIME, DATE AND PLACE AND WAS DUE TO THE CAUSE(S) STATED

SIGNATURE AND TITLE: X

40. DATE SIGNED (Mo, Day, Yr):

41. HOUR OF DEATH (24 Hrs):

42. NAME AND TITLE OF ATTENDING PHYSICIAN IF OTHER THAN CERTIFIER (Type or Print):

TO BE COMPLETED ONLY BY **MEDICAL EXAMINER OR CORONER**

43. ON THE BASIS OF EXAMINATION AND/OR INVESTIGATION, IN MY OPINION DEATH OCCURRED AT THE TIME, DATE AND PLACE AND WAS DUE TO THE CAUSE(S) STATED

SIGNATURE AND TITLE: X [redacted], MD

44. DATE SIGNED (Mo, Day, Yr): November 15, 1999

45. HOUR OF DEATH (24 Hrs): 1105

46. PRONOUNCED DEAD (Mo, Day, Yr): November [redacted], 1999

47. HOUR PRONOUNCED DEAD (24 Hrs): 1541

48. NAME AND ADDRESS OF CERTIFIER—PHYSICIAN, MEDICAL EXAMINER OR CORONER (Type or Print): [redacted], Everett, WA 98204

49. ME/CORONER FILE NUMBER: [redacted]

CAUSE OF DEATH

50. ENTER THE DISEASES, INJURIES, OR COMPLICATIONS WHICH CAUSED THE DEATH

IMMEDIATE CAUSE (Final disease or condition resulting in death)

DO NOT ENTER THE MODE OF DYING SUCH AS CARDIAC OR RESPIRATORY ARREST, SHOCK, OR HEART FAILURE. LIST ONLY ONE CAUSE ON EACH LINE. Sequentially list conditions, if any, leading to immediate cause. Enter UNDERLYING CAUSE (Disease or injury which initiated events resulting in death) LAST

	Cause	INTERVAL BETWEEN ONSET AND DEATH
A	Asphyxia	
B (DUE TO, OR AS A CONSEQUENCE OF)	Salt water drowning	
C (DUE TO, OR AS A CONSEQUENCE OF)		
D (DUE TO, OR AS A CONSEQUENCE OF)		

Field	Entry
51. OTHER SIGNIFICANT CONDITIONS—CONDITIONS CONTRIBUTING TO DEATH BUT NOT RESULTING IN THE UNDERLYING CAUSE GIVEN ABOVE	
52. AUTOPSY? (Yes / No)	Yes
53. WAS CASE REFERRED TO MEDICAL EXAMINER OR CORONER? (Yes / No)	Yes
54. ACC, SUICIDE, HOM, UNDET., OR PENDING INVEST (Specify)	Accident
55. INJURY DATE (Mo, Day, Yr)	Nov. 1999
56. HOUR OF INJURY (24 Hrs)	1103
57. DESCRIBE HOW INJURY OCCURRED	Salt water drowning
58. INJURY AT WORK? (Yes / No)	No
59. PLACE OF INJURY—AT HOME, FARM, STREET, FACTORY, OFFICE BLDG, ETC (Specify)	Puget Sound
60. LOCATION—STREET OR RFD NO., CITY/TOWN, STATE	30 yrds east of boat yard, Edmonds, WA

61. RECORD AMENDMENT (Registrar use only): ITEM / DOCUMENTARY EVIDENCE / REVIEWED BY / DATE	62. REGISTRAR SIGNATURE	63. DATE RECEIVED (Mo, Day, Yr)
	X [redacted]	NOV 18 1999

DOH 110-006 (Rev. 7/91) (formerly DSHS 9-150)

HEALTH STATISTICS & ASSESSMENT

CERTIFICATION ON BACK

DOH 01-003 (5/99)

THIS IS A CERTIFIED COPY OF THE RECORD ON FILE WITH CENTER FOR HEALTH STATISTICS. CERTIFIED COPIES MUST HAVE THE OFFICIAL SEAL.

Fig. 8.9 When you can't obtain an autopsy, you can usually obtain a copy of the death certificate which will list the cause of death.

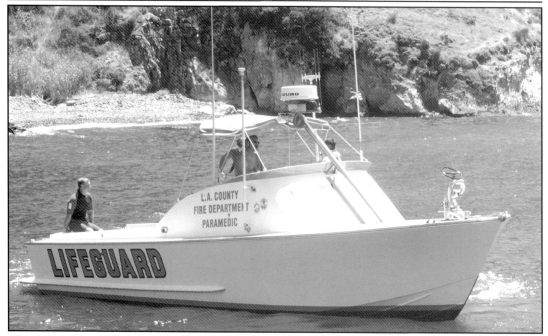

Fig. 8.10 Many lifeguards are divers and their incident reports on diving accidents can be quite helpful when they can be accessed.

ment to the Fire Department. This change in agency may limit what information you are able to obtain from the lifeguards without a subpoena.

Visiting the Library

If you need to scan back copies of the local newspaper at the library, be sure to allow yourself sufficient time to go through at least a week's worth of newspapers. This can take several hours, particularly at a library where there are a limited number of microfilm readers.

You should pay particular attention to two sections of the paper; i.e., the obituaries and the local news. It's rare for a diving accident to make the front page, unless it was a particularly dramatic accident, a very small town, or a prominent citizen.

Visiting Park Rangers

Since many beaches are part of local, state, or federal parks, you may find yourself interviewing personnel from these agencies. In most cases, they are law enforcement personnel, but will generally be more open and helpful than regular police officers. As a general rule, park rangers are oriented towards assisting visitors and tend to be cooperative. As with the lifeguards, reports or logs may exist that contain important information.

Foreign Investigations

From time to time you may be called upon to investigate a diving accident in a foreign country. These are usually the most difficult of all investigations, especially if the incident took place in a location where you do not speak the language. You'll need an interpreter who understands the language and who is knowledgeable of local customs and locations.

Employing an Interpreter

Your single most important aspect in conducting an accident investigation in a foreign country where you do not speak the language is to hire a local "interpreter." You specifically want an "interpreter" who is capable of translating speech as it occurs, rather than a "translator" who only works on written text at their own pace.

Any interpreter that you hire should be from the local area where you will conduct your investigation. This is crucial for several reasons. First, they will know and speak the local dialect. Secondly, they will be able to help you find your way around the area. Finally, they will know many of the local people, providing an introduction for you where you might otherwise be an unwelcome outsider.

You must be attuned to how the locals react to the interpreter you have employed. If you sense that the people you are visiting are hostile to the interpreter you have selected, you will need to find another interpreter quickly so that your investigation is not compromised.

You should be able to locate an interpreter by contacting the people at the local embassy. What you don't want to do is ask people from the dive store or diving company that was involved in the accident you are investigating to recommend an interpreter. There's a good chance they will recommend someone with whom they are friendly, which may compromise your investigation.

Probably the most difficult part about using an interpreter will be dealing with specific diving terminology that the interpreter doesn't know or understand. You may need to spend some time explaining the diving terms to your interpreter.

Take Anything You Think You Might Need

Unless you know that particular equipment or services are available at your destination, be sure to take anything you might think you will need. If you think you will need to dive to inspect the site, you probably won't need to take your own gear unless the diving will be particularly challenging and your own equipment will provide a higher level of safety.

A digital camera is often preferred in many resort locations, since it will eliminate the necessity for you to deal with film processing. However, almost all popular tourist destinations have one-hour film services readily available if you don't own a digital camera.

Local Customs Must be Respected

Whenever you visit a foreign country it's imperative to be sensitive to local customs, but it's even more important when you are conducting investigations. You need to establish a rapport with the local people to gain their cooperation.

You must be extremely patient as an investigator in a foreign country, since local laws and traditions will inevitably be quite different from the way things are at home. You may need to re-visit government offices multiple times before you get to see the person who can release or locate the information that you need. For example, on the island of Cozumel in Mexico, only the firemen can move a dead body and there is only one fire station. Their reports are recorded by hand in a ledger and they have no photocopy machine.

A bottle of tequila can provide the lubricant needed to get the officer in charge to have his secretary type up an official copy of the report on a diving fatality. The custom of "mordita" (the bite) should be viewed neither as bribery or corruption. It is simply the way things are done. To someone unfamiliar with the concept of tipping, it might seem strange to pay someone an additional amount to do the job expected of him. In much the same way, "mordita" should be viewed as a tip, a custom, or the way things are done. Just be sure that you are discrete about how you handle such things and check with your interpreter to be sure that what you intend to do fits within local customs.

Bureaucracy Is the Same the World Over

Getting information released by government agencies can be difficult anywhere, but even more so in a foreign country. Some countries do not have organizations like the Coast Guard, so it may take time to determine who would have handled the response to a particular incident.

In a death case, the divemaster or boat crew may even be arrested in some countries, until they are cleared of homicide charges. Don't make any presumptions if this occurs, as it may be purely a routine procedure.

People May Tell You What They Think You Want to Hear

In some foreign countries, particularly if you are dealing with a native boat crew that is not well educated or extremely poor, there is a tendency for these people to tell you what they think it is you want to hear. It is extremely important in these circumstances to explain to them up front that it is important for them to tell you only what they know to be true without making any assumptions. They also must understand that it is appropriate for them to admit that they don't know the answer to some questions. You must be prepared to recognize that some of the interviews you conduct under these circumstances may not have much value when it comes to producing your report.

Medical Records are Confidential in Most Countries

Just as they are in the U.S., medical records are confidential in most countries in the world. While you should always make the attempt to collect any information that you can, you can expect that you will be denied access to hospital records in most countries.

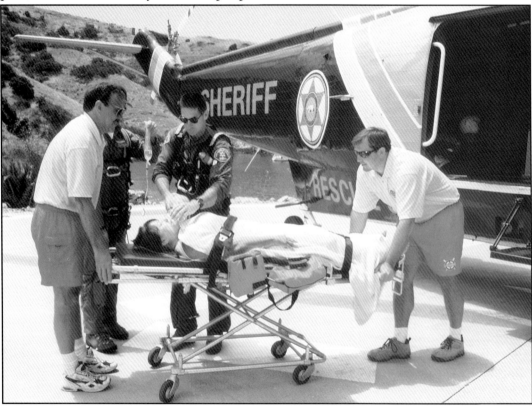

Fig. 8.11 Paramedics' reports and medical records are considered confidential almost everywhere, and you will not be able to obtain these unless you are in law enforcement or have a subpoena.

Case History – Commercial Oilfield Diving

A diving bell owned by a large commercial diving firm was sent ashore for maintenance when a job it was on ended. One of the technicians, who worked on the bell, pulled all of the Lexan® viewports, cleaned their sealing surfaces, and reinstalled the ports.

Diving bell ports are a bit unusual compared to viewports in decompression chambers that remain on the deck. What makes them different is that a diving bell port must seal in two directions. As the bell descends, and the pressure outside exceeds the pressure inside, the port must seal the bell shut against the mounting external pressure. Conversely, as the bell returns to the surface after the dive, it must hold the pressure inside it constant, even as the pressure outside decreases.

Ports are sealed in the steel hull of diving bells using rubber o-ring seals. There are actually two o-rings for each port, one to seal during the descent to the bottom with the external pressure, and one to seal during the ascent to the surface with the internal pressure. Unfortunately, the technician installed an incorrectly sized o-ring in one of the ports. To further compound the problem, when a big job came up unexpectedly, the bell was sent back out into the field as part of a saturation diving system, without the required testing.

On the first dive back in the field, the bell worked properly during the descent, when the internal o-ring sealed against the hull. However, at the end of the dive, when the divers closed the internal hatch and attempted to get a seal, i.e., to hold the internal pressure in the bell constant by sealing the hatch with pressure, the port began to leak past the o-ring.

Because the port was leaking at its highest point, it wasn't apparent to the divers inside the bell where the leak was occurring. Although there was no immediate danger to the divers, the supervisor wanted to get the bell back up to the surface because the weather topside was deteriorating.

The supervisor tried repeatedly to blow heli-ox gas into the bell in an attempt to achieve a proper seal, but without success. Finally, with the weather growing more threatening, and a diminishing supply of breathing gas aboard the support vessel, the supervisor made the decision to bring the bell rapidly to the surface with the hope of getting the divers into the saturation complex topside before too much pressure was lost.

During the ascent, the leak from the port increased and the internal pressure inside the diving bell rapidly diminished. One of the divers died during the explosive decompression, while the other suffered a severe case of decompression sickness. It wasn't until the bell was subsequently examined following the dive, that the mistake the technician had made was discovered.

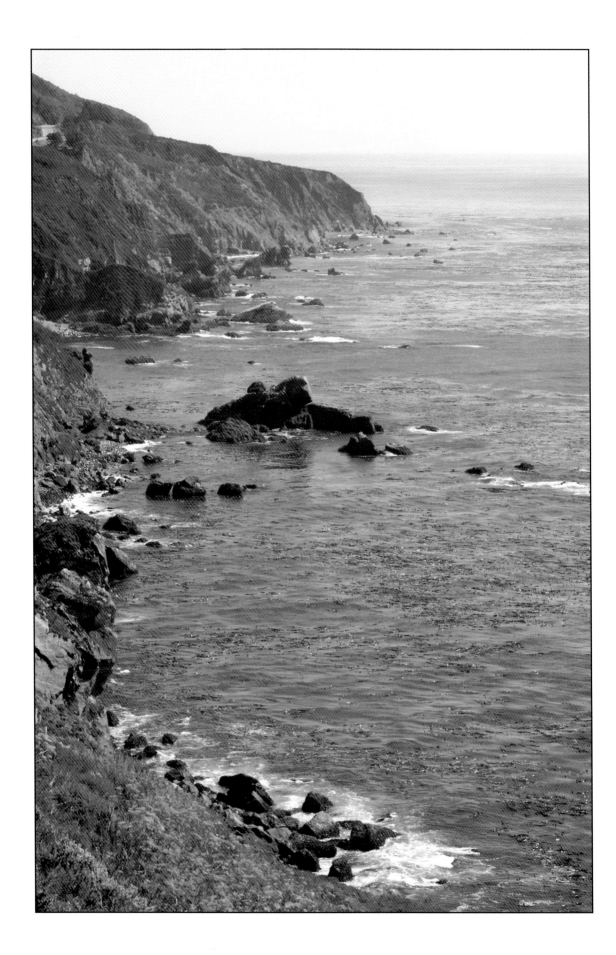

Chapter 9
Inspecting the Dive Accident Site

While it is rare for a diving accident investigator to find the need to actually make a dive to inspect a dive site, occasionally this is essential. In most cases, a topside inspection of the site is more than sufficient, but if the site has unusual features or if the accident was especially serious and the investigator is unfamiliar with the site, it may be appropriate. As an investigator, it will usually be clear to you which course of action is best.

Before you visit a site, be sure to check out any information resources, such as the NOAA weather pages on the Internet, to determine historic conditions at the time of the accident. If the site is a popular one, or one that NOAA regularly monitors, such as Avalon Harbor at Catalina Island, you may be able to obtain detailed information on the conditions on the day of the incident.

While most of what is covered in this chapter will be applicable primarily to sport diving, there are many issues that will be relevant to professional or commercial diving incidents as well.

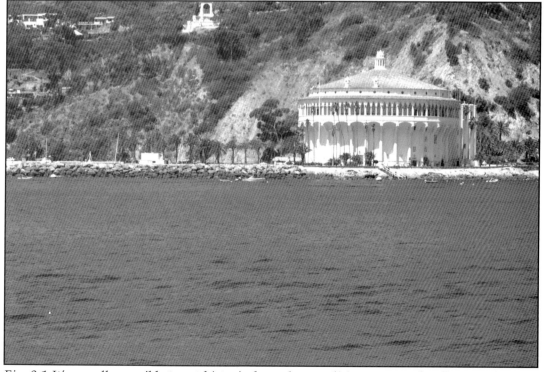

Fig. 9.1 It's usually possible to get historical weather conditions on popular dive sites like the harbor at Avalon on Catalina Island.

General Environmental Factors That Affect All Diving

Environmental factors often play a big role in diving accidents. Factors such as kelp, surf, ice, water temperature and other issues may be a contributing cause to a diving accident, although they will rarely be the direct cause of the accident. In most cases, a lack of training or experience, a procedural mistake by the diver, or a failure by an instructor to follow established procedures will be more important than any environmental factor.

Kelp

Kelp is a layman's term that may be applied to a variety of large marine algaes. In actuality, there are many different types of aquatic plants that are not "kelp," as well as several specific species that are commonly referred to as kelp.

In California, when most divers refer to "kelp" they are referring to *Macrocystis pyrifera*, which is a type of kelp that may grow from the bottom to the surface in water depths as deep as 100 FSW. However, there are other types of kelp in California, such as "bull kelp," that has thicker stalks, tends to live in deeper wa-

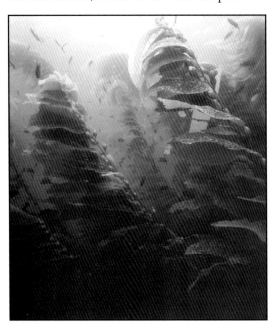

9.2 A properly trained diver should have no difficulty moving through kelp.

ters, and grows up to 60 feet in length, but the plants are usually widely spaced.

Although you will frequently read articles about diving accidents that attribute the cause of a diver's death to entanglement in "thick kelp," a properly trained or supervised diver should never die due to entanglement in kelp. With proper training, any diver should be able to maneuver through thick aquatic plants.

It's almost always easier for a diver to swim through kelp underwater than it is to swim across a thick mat of kelp on the surface. On the surface, it's possible for a diver to swim across the top of a kelp bed by using a technique known as "kelp crawling," where the diver reaches out and grabs armfuls of kelp and pulls them to his chest.

Kelp that becomes entangled in a diver's gear can be difficult to break by pulling it lengthwise, but by bending each individual stalk tightly, the kelp will snap. This action is not intuitive and a panicked diver is unlikely to think of this.

In cases where a diver is found unconscious in thick kelp, it's usually because they did not have proper training in how to swim across the kelp on the surface and then became fatigued and panicked.

Kelp is not a permanent fixture at any dive site because kelp beds can die due to pollution, a lack of nutrients, overgrazing by animals that eat kelp, and changes in water temperature. Kelp beds can also be devastated by strong storms that tear up the plants. If you do not visit the site until weeks after the incident took place, it may look entirely different than it did on the day that the accident took place.

Currents

The maximum speed at which most divers in good physical condition can swim through the water is one knot, and few divers can sustain this type of effort for any length of time. For this reason, a well-trained diver will always plan his

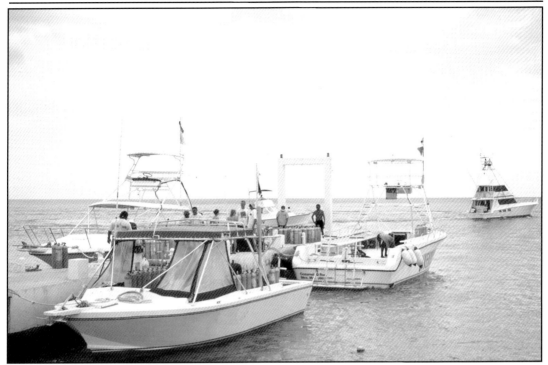

Fig. 9.3 The island of Cozumel is popular for diving, but known for its strong currents.

dive into the current, so that he can return to the boat with the current.

Most sport diving boats will deploy a "current line" when operating in areas where there is a current. The current line consists of several hundred feet of polypropylene line with a float attached to the end. The line is connected to the boat so that divers who surface down current behind the boat can pull themselves back to the vessel along the line.

Currents, however, can and do change, sometimes unexpectedly. This is especially true at offshore locations.

Along the west coast of the U.S. the primary current flow is from north to south. However, when there is a hurricane off the Baja coast, the current flow sometimes reverses itself. This can be disconcerting to a new diver who encounters this change for the first time.

Along the east coast, the Gulf Stream is a powerful current that moves in and out from shore, and travels at tremendous speed. Diving along the east coast is usually planned with the Gulf Stream in mind.

Currents typically pose a problem for scuba divers when they are swept away from their entry point or the boat. In most cases, the boat operator will be aware that there are currents and will be watching for divers who surface down current and who might be having difficulty returning to the boat. Savvy divers typically carry signalling devices with them so that they can signal the boat to pick them up if they are down current.

In most cases, when a diver is swept away by a current, the diver is in no immediate danger, unless he panics. However, divers have been lost at sea and died under these circumstances, but this is rare.

Most currents move horizontally through the water. There are some locations in the world, such as Palau in the South Pacific, and Cozumel in the Caribbean where there are strong "downdraft" currents, that can actually force a diver down into deep water. In these situations, the diver may be forced to inflate his BC fully at depth and/or drop weights in order to return to the surface.

Currents can place a lot of drag on a commercial diver's hose and can greatly increase the amount of effort a diver must expend to work. It is not uncommon for a commercial diver to tie his hose off to a nearby structure to eliminate the pull on his hose by the current. If this procedure is used, the diver must use a knot that will untie instantly if needed.

One of the problems for a commercial diver working in a current is to have a novice tender handling the hose. An inexperienced tender may interpret the pull placed on the hose by the current as a "request" from the diver for additional hose. Putting too much slack hose into the water can cause the diver's hose to become "fouled" (caught) on underwater obstructions.

Tides

In certain parts of the world, the effect of tides can have a dramatic influence on diving operations. This is particularly true in areas like the Pacific Northwest, where the tides can greatly affect the volume and speed of the water passing between the narrow passages of the islands.

Most diving in areas of large tidal change must be planned around the ebb and flow of the tide, with the bulk of the diving taking place just prior to or at slack tide.

Tides can substantially alter the look of a beach and the access to it. Tides may uncover rocks or other structures that make beach access difficult.

Thermoclines

Thermoclines are layers of water, at different temperatures, that occur in large bodies of water. These temperature variations can be quite dramatic and may affect underwater visibility and other aspects of the dive.

Typically, the water will be warmer above the thermocline than below it. Thermoclines can occur at any depth, but most seem to occur at depths below 20-30 feet.

Colder waters tend to be clearer than the warmer water layers. It is not uncommon to descend through a warmer layer of reduced visibility and "break through" to a layer of crystal clear cold water.

Thermoclines can interfere with wireless underwater communication systems that are frequently used by public safety divers and diving scientists.

Underwater Visibility

Visibility can be a major contributing factor in a diving accident for any number of reasons. While the normal visibility in air in most locations during the day may be miles, the best underwater visibility is usually no more than 200 feet. In some locations, the "average" underwater visibility may be no more than 10-20 feet. What this means is that if the underwater visibility is 20 feet and an object is 30 feet away, you won't see it.

Most divers are a bit uncomfortable when the visibility is reduced to less than five or six feet, and this is particularly true for novice divers. When the visibility is reduced to one foot or less, conditions are described as "zero visibility." Any type of scuba diving becomes more hazardous in reduced visibility.

Some commercial divers regularly work in zero visibility conditions, particularly divers who work in harbors or other similar locations. Even though these divers are accustomed to this type of work, there is an increased risk for these professionals, too.

The underwater visibility can vary greatly with the season. For example, during winter months in the midwest, the underwater visibility in most lakes improves dramatically as plankton (microscopic plants and animals) and algae in the water dies as the water becomes colder. High winds blowing across the ocean can cause "upwelling" in certain locations, bringing cold, nutrient-rich water to the surface, causing plankton to "bloom," reducing visibility.

Low Temperatures

Diving in cold water is generally more hazardous than diving in warm water. To dive in cold water, the diver must wear heavier insulation, which restricts movement and increases the diver's work load. Gloves must be worn and these reduce manual dexterity.

The temperature ranges at most popular dive sites are generally well known for a given time of year. If the dive was for recreation and the diver was using a dive computer, it will generally be possible to determine the exact temperature during any phase of the dive where the accident occurred. Most newspapers published in coastal cities will also list surface ocean temperatures on their weather page. Historical and real-time ocean temperatures from buoys located at sea are also available from NOAA (National Oceanic and Atmospheric Administration) on the Internet.

Altitude

High altitude diving presents a special set of circumstances that can cause problems for the diver. Dives at altitude are made in fresh water and at reduced atmospheric pressure.

In seawater, 33 feet of depth equals one atmosphere (14.7 p.s.i.) of pressure, while in fresh water, one atmosphere equals 34 feet of depth. At altitude, reduced barometric pressure requires more decompression than equivalent dives made at sea level. In addition, when a diver first arrives at altitude, this change in pressure must be taken into account in decompression calculations. This can be done using decompression tables specifically designed for use at altitude, although most dive computers today will allow the user to adjust them for altitude use.

Surf

Surf can be a serious problem for recreational divers who are attempting to enter or exit the water from the beach.

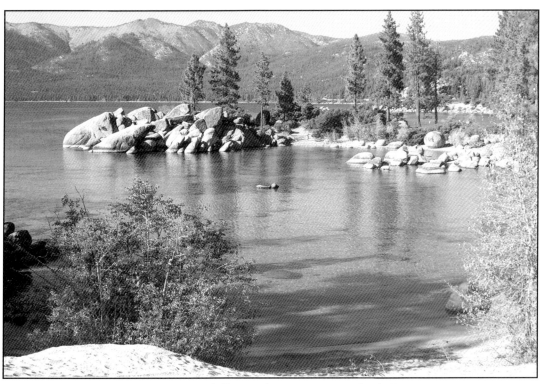

Fig. 9.4 Diving at altitude requires different decompression calculations.

Divers who have no surf training and attempt to enter the water through surf may experience problems in this environment. Experienced divers who have had the proper training are able to make entries and exits from beaches where waves are in excess of six feet. However, you should be in exceptionally good physical condition to attempt to dive in this type of environment.

Most divers who have problems in surf make the mistake of stopping in the zone where the waves are breaking, usually due to some type of equipment problem or fatigue. This action can have undesirable consequences.

Many beaches only have high surf on an occasional basis, while others have a consistent "break." Be aware that as an investigator you may not be viewing the site under the same conditions that were present when the accident took place.

Overhead Environments

Any environment in which a diver cannot make a direct ascent to the surface is considered an "overhead environment." Overhead environments are considered much more dangerous than the "typical" open water diving environment. These situations include diving under ice, penetration into shipwrecks, and cave diving. Staged decompression dives are considered to take place in a "virtual overhead environment," since the diver must complete his planned steps before he ascends to the surface.

Unless you are fully qualified for the particular type of overhead environment in which the accident took place, you must not attempt to dive the site. In many cases, it will also be difficult for you to perform a proper gear inspection or know whether the correct procedures were followed in these situations unless you are experienced in this type of diving. In this situation, you will probably need to hire an instructor with expertise in this area to assist you. If you are investigating the

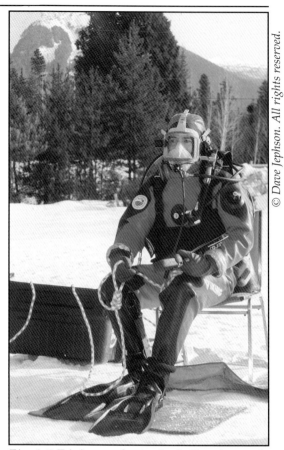

© Dave Jephson. All rights reserved.

Fig. 9.5 Diving under ice is challenging and requires special gear and training.

case on behalf of an attorney, you'll need to get approval before you take this step.

If you must hire another person to assist you in a particular specialty area, you'll need to ensure that they understand exactly what you want them to do and that they must hold the information regarding the case confidential. You should have them sign a confidentiality agreement so that they appreciate the seriousness of their involvement.

Ice

Diving under the ice presents multiple hazards. Aside from the problems with the diver's own thermal protection, there can also be problems with equipment, such as regulators, that "freeze" at low temperatures due to water or moisture in the unit. A regulator that "freezes" in the open position is in a condition known as a "free flow," and will lead to a rapid depletion of the diver's air supply.

The other major hazard in ice diving is in losing one's way back to the entry/exit point. Most ice diving is done in lakes, where an access hole is cut through the ice. Proper procedures call for each diver who enters the water to be tethered to topside by a safety line that is tended by a person topside. If the line is accidentally cut, comes untied, or was not used in the first place, it can be impossible to find the exit point.

If you are unable to visit the site soon after the accident took place, you may find that the access hole that was used to make the dive has frozen over and is no longer identifiable. Worse yet, if you are unable to visit the site until the season has changed there may be no ice present, making it difficult to get an accurate idea of what conditions were like at the time of the event.

Wrecks

Shipwrecks are extremely popular with sport divers. They make interesting dives by themselves, and usually attract a variety of marine life. Some divers also collect artifacts from wrecks, which may or may not be legal, depending on the location, age, and ownership of the wreck.

Most recreational divers content themselves with exploring the exterior of wrecks and avoid entering them. Technical divers, however, frequently enter or "penetrate" shipwrecks in order to collect artifacts, take photographs or video, or simply pursue the challenge of exploring the most intricate passages of a deep wreck.

Many shipwrecks are covered with fishing nets or monofilament line that is difficult to see and that can snag a diver's equipment. Prudent wreck divers carry knives and other cutting devices to deal with these nuisances.

Penetration wreck diving can be extremely hazardous. The interior of most

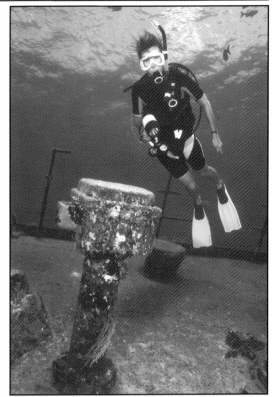

Fig. 9.6 Shipwrecks provide an enticement for divers. Wreck penetration can be dangerous.

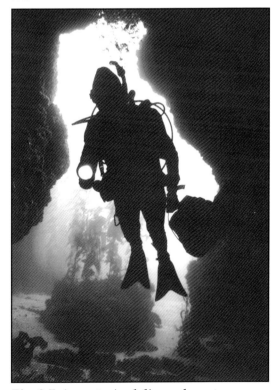

Fig. 9.7 An untrained diver who enters a cave is courting disaster.

shipwrecks are without light and the passageways are layered with fine organic silt that is easily stirred up by a careless fin kick. When this silt becomes suspended, the visibility inside the wreck may be instantly reduced to zero, and it may take hours for the silt to settle out.

Caverns and Caves

A cavern is a natural underwater rock formation that a diver can enter that will prevent a direct ascent to the surface, but in which a diver always can see natural light. By comparison, in a cave, not only can the diver not make a direct ascent, but the diver also can go beyond the zone of natural light.

Cavern diving can be enjoyed by almost any diver with a minimum of additional training and the addition of no more equipment than a dive light. By contrast, cave diving requires extensive additional training and a vast amount of extra equipment.

Cave diving is considered much more dangerous than cavern diving, since a diver may explore hundreds or even thousands of feet inside a cave. There are many cave diving deaths every year, most of which are attributed to a lack of proper training, or a failure to follow the correct procedures.

Deaths that occur within a cave re-quire a specialized investigation. The exact distance to the cave mouth must be ascertained. Detailed attention must be given to the "rules" of cave diving and whether they were followed.

The simplest equipment failure that on a standard recreational dive would be only a nuisance can result in a fatality in a cave dive. Visibility, with and without the bottom stirred up, needs to be determined. The possibility of current reversal also needs to be explored. Unless you are intimately familiar with cave diving this type of investigation should be referred to someone else.

Deep Sites that Require Staged Decompression Following the Dive

At any dive site where the depth exceeds 130 FSW, there is a good chance that the diving will require a series of decompression stops. Planned decompression diving is usually considered outside the realm of sport diving and part of technical diving. It may require extensive extra equipment and planning to be done properly.

There is a small but growing group of technical divers who are routinely making dives in the 150-250 FSW depth range. Some are making dives much deeper than this. The investment in time and

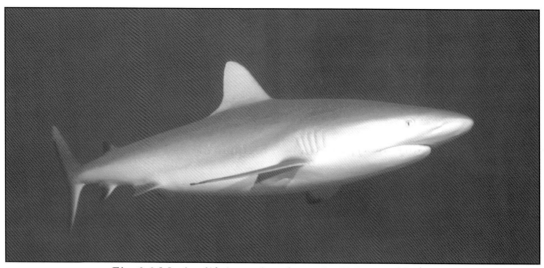

Fig. 9.8 Marine life is rarely a factor in diving accidents.

Risk Recognition for Divers and Diving Professionals

Most dive operations, whether they are recreational or commercial, are usually dependent on chartered vessels to provide topside support for their diving activities. In most cases, if you are dealing with a U.S. Coast Guard licensed captain, the boat will be operated and maintained in a responsible fashion. The typical boat captain finds the risk of losing his "ticket" (license) too high a gamble to run a shoddy operation.

However, as the person who chartered the vessel, it's your duty to make sure that the vessel is run responsibly, and to bring it to the attention of the captain if you see things that you find unacceptable. When you first board a vessel, be sure to check for life jackets, fire extinguishers, an operable radio, and other safety equipment. Take a good look around to be sure that the vessel appears to be in good repair and make note of any conditions that may be a problem. Don't be afraid to speak to the captain, if you are concerned about any aspects of the operation.

---

money to conduct these types of dives places it outside the realm of the average recreational diver.

Marine Life

Marine life is rarely a factor in a diving accident, although the potential for an injury or fatality caused by marine life almost always exists. Thousands of people participate in scuba diving each year without encountering dangerous marine life.

Probably the only creatures in the ocean that regularly are responsible for the death of a diver are sharks, and even these incidents are extremely rare. While shark attacks are known to occur in all seas worldwide, they are more common in colder waters, particularly near sites where marine mammals (such as seals and sea lions) are common.

Even when sharks do attack, the injuries sustained by most divers are not fatal. Each type of shark has a characteristic shape to its teeth and experts are frequently able to identify the type of shark from bite marks and whole teeth, or even fragments, left in the wounds.

It is important to point out that although sharks attack swimmers with some regularity, shark attacks on scuba divers are much less common. As a result, when investigating a "shark attack"

death always consider the possibility that wounds attributed to sharks occurred after death had already taken place.

Beaches

Seasonal variations in surf can also have a dramatic impact on the configuration of a beach site. For example, on the west coast of the U.S., winter storms and high surf take much of the sand away from many beaches, exposing rocks that are not normally visible during the summer. During the summer months, the sand accumulates on the beaches again, changing the appearance of the beach dramatically.

Day to Night Changes

If you are investigating a diving accident that took place at night, you will probably want to visit the site after dark to see how the site appears once the sun goes down. This is particularly important if the accident involved night diving that took place off a beach. If possible, photograph the site during the day and at night.

Diving the Site

As previously mentioned, in most cases there is little need for the investigator to personally dive the site to perform an inspection. This is especially true if

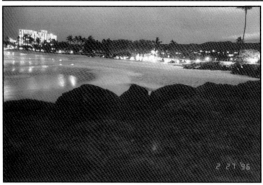

Fig. 9.9 If the accident took place at night, be sure to visit the site at night to see how it differs from the way it appears during daylight hours.

the accident took place in an area where the investigator is familiar with the general conditions. However, if the case is a serious one, and it appears there will be litigation regarding the incident, it is usually important to dive the site to give the attorneys who will be working on the case a detailed picture of the site. Under these circumstances, there is no substitute for high quality photographs and video, as well as water temperature readings and accurate depth measurements.

In commercial diving accidents it may be impractical for the investigator to dive the site, particularly in situations where the water is extremely deep, conditions are hazardous, or construction work is ongoing.

Photographing the Site Underwater

While video is very helpful in getting a broad overview of a dive site, still photographs are quite useful for highlighting particular features of a site that may need to be studied in greater detail. There is a strong case for this if the accident took place on a shipwreck or other site that has distinctive features.

Photographs should be taken from as many angles as possible so that it is possible to see features that may not be visible from a single view. In addition, you should always attempt to include some

type of item in the photograph that will provide a sense of scale. A plastic ruler is not usually practical for this purpose, as some plastic rulers will float. Instead, you may want to use a brightly colored diving weight, a dive knife, or some other easily identifiable object.

Whenever photo or video is shot with the potential that it may be used in court, the images should always be "date-stamped" by the camera if possible. Since the features of a dive site may change over time, this may become important.

Video

Video is a powerful tool that can be used to convey information that is not easily communicated in still photographs. If you need to show the path that a diver took through a wreck underwater, there is no substitute for a video recording.

Although it is relatively easy to edit video using a personal computer, you should do no editing of the video you have taken, unless you have been specifically instructed to do so. If a video is edited, there is usually a question in court as to what might have been deliberately edited out of the recording.

Inspections of Recreational Sites

Some recreational sites are the scene of frequent accidents, not because they are particularly dangerous, but because they are so heavily used by instructors and divers. For example, Catalina Island off the coast of Los Angeles is one of the more benign sites in Southern California, but it is such a popular diving destination that several accidents take place there each year.

More challenging dive sites also take their toll of advanced and technical divers with some regularity. Multiple deaths have occurred on the wreck of the sunken Italian liner *Andrea Doria* off the east coast. Shrouded with fishing nets at great depth, and in a state of decay, the *"Doria"* presents a challenge even to the most experienced technical diver.

Whenever you are inspecting a shore based dive site that is not familiar to you, take your time and look around very carefully. It's helpful if you can obtain a chart before your visit so you understand the bottom terrain. Sometimes there will be more detailed maps prepared by local users of the site available from dive stores or in dive guide books.

If there are no detailed maps or sketches of the site, you may want to make your own. It's helpful to have a fiberglass measuring tape with you to note the distances from various features of the site to each other. For example, if there is a telephone on shore, note the distance relative to the stairs used for entry, or the distance from parking lot to the pier. You'll also want to note the distances from the site to wherever emergency service providers were dispatched, so that you can compare this to response times.

Using your handheld GPS, you should record the location of key features of the site to answer any questions that may arise later. While there is some variability in GPS readings, this can be an invaluable tool in creating a detailed report.

If there were unusual environmental conditions at the site when the accident occurred, you should try to visit the location under the same type of conditions.

Stairs to Entry Point

At some dive locations, there are concrete stairs that have been installed as an entry point into the water. Such stairs are frequently slippery and are the cause of numerous falls. When a diver is fully geared up, with a tank on his back, a fall can be a dangerous accident.

Sites Where Sport Diving Accidents Occur Frequently

The following locations are some popular sites that have seen a high number of diving accidents. As stated previ-

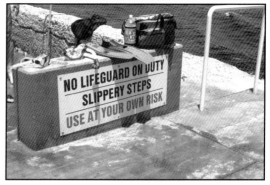

Fig. 9.10 Stairs that enter the water may be quite slippery and produce frequent falls.

ously, these are extremely popular dive sites and since a great deal of diving is done at these spots, accidents are to be expected.

Catalina Island, California

Catalina Island is a favorite diving location not only because it offers very good diving, but also due to its proximity to Southern California and Los Angeles in particular. However, despite its clear water and generally calm conditions, Catalina is still considered a cold water diving location with water temperatures in the low to mid 60s most of the year.

The dive sites at the town of Avalon, towards the eastern end of the island, see some of the most consistent use by divers. There is an underwater park adjacent to the Casino that provides easy access to the water via a set of stone stairs that lead directly into the sea. This is a popular training site for instructors to use, and many groups pick this area for their open water training.

Farnsworth Bank is an advanced dive site that can only be reached by boat. It is an underwater pinnacle located several miles off the ocean side of the island in deep water that extends beyond traditional sport diving depths. Divers have been injured and/or died at this location when they have mistakenly gone too deep. The clear water and rapid drop-off here make it relatively easy for a careless or poorly trained diver to get in trouble.

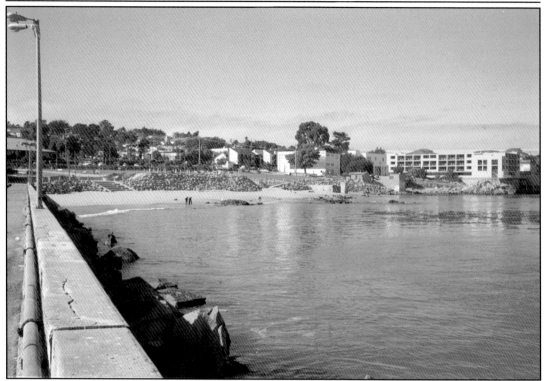

Fig. 9.11 The breakwater at the harbor in Monterey, California is an extremely popular dive site for training and other activities.

Monterey, California

Monterey is a common diving destination for sport divers from all over Northern and Southern California. The water in Monterey is generally colder, rougher, and not as clear as the water in Southern California. However, for many new divers, Monterey is their first experience in ocean diving.

One of the most well-liked training sites in Monterey is the beach directly adjacent to the parking lot at the breakwater at the harbor. Although the water here is normally calm, it is still a challenging environment due to the low temperature and frequently low visibility.

There are usually one or two diving fatalities each year in Monterey.

Florida

Both coasts of Florida see heavy traffic from divers throughout the year, at many different sites. Sites such as West Palm Beach on the east coast and Panama City on the panhandle are used for scuba instruction, as well as by many certified divers.

The Florida Keys are frequently visited by tourists as well as residents from the state of Florida. Diving is available throughout the keys, starting at John Pennekamp Coral Reef State Park in Key Largo and extending all the way down to Key West.

Florida has numerous freshwater springs, particularly in the northern part of the state, that are used by divers for both training and exploration. There have been numerous accidents from untrained divers entering the underwater caves that are located at many of these springs.

Hawaii

Hawaii is one of the most popular tourist destinations in the world, with its pleasant weather and warm, clear waters. A tremendous number of divers learn to dive in Hawaii. Many people also enroll in a scuba experience program that offers the opportunity to dive under the direct supervision of a diving instructor, but provides no certification for independent diving.

Diving accidents take place in Hawaii simply due to the sheer number of divers who visit the state.

Lake Travis, Austin, Texas

Lake Travis is a large, freshwater lake several miles outside Austin, Texas. It is regularly used as a training site for divers from all over Texas. Easy access and scenic campgrounds make Lake Travis a destination for divers who enjoy spending the weekend outdoors.

Although Lake Travis is an attractive lake in a pleasant setting, the visibility in the lake is usually quite low due to silt, and the water is cold.

Cozumel, Mexico

With its close proximity to the United States, Cozumel is a common diving destination for visitors who want to dive in warm water, but want a relatively inexpensive vacation. Located off the coast of

mainland Mexico, Cozumel is a tropical island with coral reefs and swift currents.

A fair number of diving accidents occur in Cozumel simply due to its close proximity to the U.S. and the sheer number of visiting divers who travel there.

Inspecting Dive Boats and Other Vessels

While only a few accidents directly involve dive boats injuring divers, a great deal of diving takes place from boats. If the accident involved a boat dive, and the injured diver was brought back aboard the vessel for first aid, you should look at the boat, if possible, to understand what took place once the diver was recovered from the water.

Layout of deck

Record the layout of the deck and note the position of the entry "doors," the location of the ladder, visibility from the "bridge" and other key features. If there are critical issues regarding visibility of a

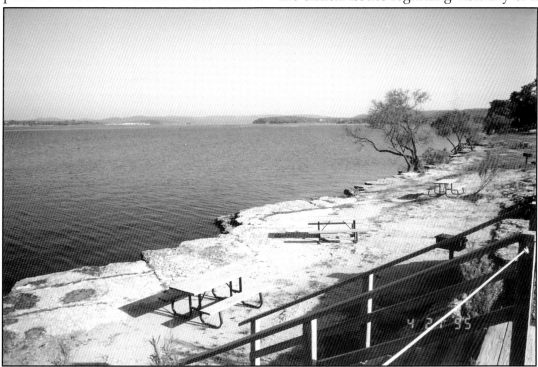

Fig. 9.12 Lake Travis, near Austin, Texas, is a picturesque setting in the country. It is a popular training site for divers from all over Texas.

diver from the boat or resuscitation of the diver, be sure to do a detailed drawing.

Obtain a Copy of the Ship's log

If at all possible, you'll want to photocopy the ship's log from the day of the incident, especially if it contains critical times, names, locations, or other information. You may not always be able to obtain the log, or the log may be poorly filled out, but you should make the effort to obtain this document if possible.

Location of Emergency Equipment

Note the location of any emergency gear that is aboard the boat, particularly if it was used in responding to the accident. Identify and locate the oxygen kit, backboard, first aid kit, rescue buoys, and any other similar items.

Be sure to note the condition of the emergency gear. Check the oxygen cylinder to see whether it is full and carefully examine the oxygen mask. Examine the

inventory of the first aid kit to see what items are missing.

Obtain a Copy of the Manifest

The manifest is a document (list) that shows all of the people who were on the boat on any particular day. While larger boats will normally have a formal manifest, particularly if you are dealing with a Coast Guard inspected vessel with a licensed captain, smaller boats may not be able to produce a formal document. You may need to compile your own list of passengers from individual documents the captain holds.

Inspecting the Hull and Propeller of a Vessel

Sometimes divers have been struck by the very boat from which they have been diving. When this occurs, and you're the investigator, you'll usually need to make a dive underneath the boat to photograph the hull, its features, and the props. You'll also need to take measurements of the

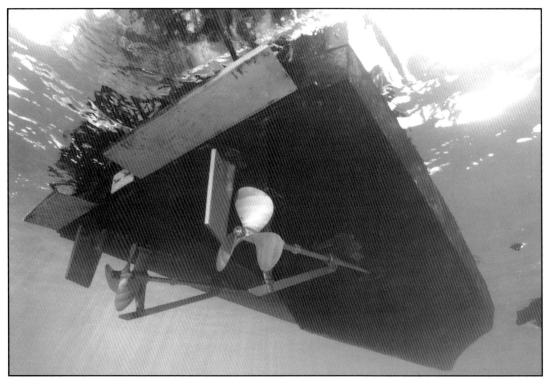

Fig. 9.13 If a diver is struck by the moving props of a boat, the results can be lethal. Of course, any impact with other features of the vessel can be damaging if the vessel is moving.

dimensions on the hull if you are unable to obtain any builder's drawings of the boat from the owner. Depending on the type of injury and how it occurred, some of the measurements that should be taken underwater include:

- Diameter of the prop/pitch of the prop
- Distance from the center of the prop to the stern
- Depth of the propeller and/or outdrive below the waterline
- Width of the boat (beam) at the stern along the bottom of the hull
- Distance from the edge of the blade of the prop to the edge of the hull along either side.
- Dimensions of any through-hull penetrators, such as depth transducers, seawater intakes, etc.
- Dimensions of any portion of the ladder or swim-step that is below the waterline.
- Depth that the ladder or swim-step extends below the waterline

From these measurements, a simple drawing of the hull and its features should be made. You may also want to shoot video of the vessel underway while you are submerged. Obviously, you must have good visibility to do this and you must take extreme care not to be struck by the boat yourself.

You should photograph and record your observations of the captain's view from the wheelhouse or other steering stations on the boat. This is especially important if the boat was maneuvering to pick up a diver by backing down, or operating in reverse for any reason. In this type of circumstance, you may also need to consider the captain's height and the direction the boat was facing when the incident took place. If it was a bright, sunny day, and the stern of the vessel was pointing into the sun, it may have been difficult for the skipper to see divers in

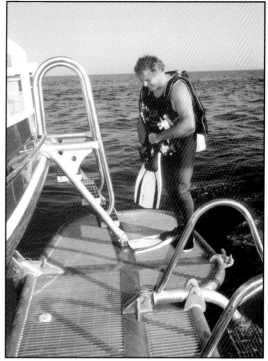

Fig. 9.14 If a tank falls out of a back-pack on the swimstep of a dive boat, anyone below it can be seriously injured.

the water. You should record the distance of the line of sight from the helmsman's position to the back deck and whether the operator was wearing any type of corrective eyewear (or needed corrective eyewear).

Divers have also been injured when a tank has fallen out of a backpack onto a diver below on the ladder or swimstep. You should make measurements from the deck to the swimstep and to calculate the geometry of the relationship between the two.

Case History – Recreational Diving

A manufacturer of buoyancy compensators issued a recall for a series of defective power inflators. The end caps on the mechanisms were not properly designed and came unscrewed too easily. Once the end cap fell off, the inflator would auto-inflate the BC. Although no incidents had occurred underwater, the manufacturer issued a recall and replaced the inflators.

An individual who was aware of the recall purchased a BC with one of the defective inflators and staged an accident at a tropical diving resort. The diver claimed that the cap came off the power inflator and the BC sent him rocketing to the surface. Following the dive, he claimed he developed decompression sickness on the flight home from the resort. The diver and his wife filed a suit against the manufacturer as well as the dive store who sold the equipment.

The equipment was examined by an expert for the defense and there were no outward signs of any problem. Tests were run by the defense with an identical BC and the same design inflator, under the same conditions (at the same site) as the alleged accident. The accident could not be duplicated, but since it could not be proven that the accident had been staged, the case proceeded. The plaintiffs produced a video to support their claim.

As the case developed, the plaintiff claimed that he could no longer work, that he was unable to engage in his favorite sports and hobbies, and that his mental capacity was diminished. Just prior to the deposition of one of the defense experts it was discovered that the plaintiff was, in fact, working as an expert in an entirely unrelated case, despite the fact he said he could not work. During his deposition in the unrelated case he testified that he worked full time, despite his testimony in the dive case to the contrary. In addition, it was subsequently discovered that the plaintiff had signed a contract to work at an institution very close to one of his favorite skiing sites during the period where he was claiming complete disability. Other witnesses who knew him also testified that he had been seen skiing.

The case proceeded to trial and a defense verdict was rendered. Subsequent to the original trial, the plaintiff's medical insurance carrier sued the plaintiff for false disability claims.

Notes:

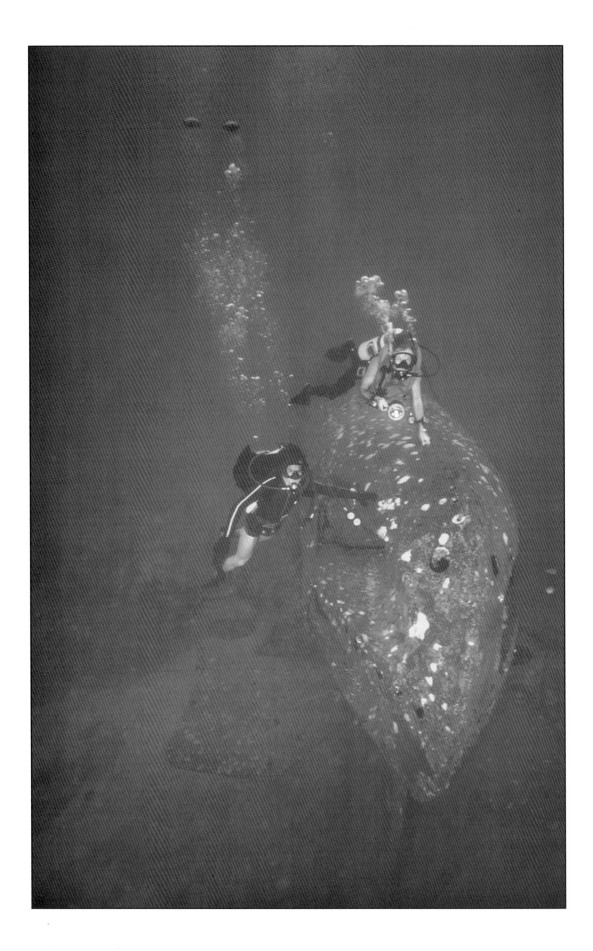

Chapter 10
Non-Diving Accidents

As a diving accident investigator, you may be called upon to investigate accidents and events that didn't occur in the water, but did involve diving equipment or happen in a diving setting. These types of accidents and incidents are quite common and some of them can produce serious injuries. Examples of such accidents and incidents include oxygen fires, compressor accidents, eye injuries, and sexual harassment.

Oxygen Fires

With the increasing use of nitrox and the prevalence of technical diving, oxygen fires have become a serious concern in recreational diving. In commercial diving, oxygen fires have always been a threat, but their occurrence has been rare.

Whenever high-pressure oxygen is used, all of the components of the diving system must be cleaned following special procedures to ensure the removal of all hydrocarbons. In addition, all of the components of the system that come into contact with high pressure oxygen must be oxygen compatible and must be lubricated with oxygen safe lubricants.

Oxygen fires are probably most common in situations where high-pressure oxygen is being used to create specialized gas mixtures. If there are any hydrocarbons in the gas system the potential for a fire is high. Flammable materials usually enter the system through the use of improper lubricants or when compressed air from an oil lubricated compressor is introduced into a system that was previously cleaned for oxygen use.

On the recreational side, oxygen fires have occurred in dive stores mixing gas for nitrox use due to the contamination of the store's own system. At least one sport diver has had an oxygen fire occur when the equipment on his back ignited, probably caused by a combination of a hydrocarbon contaminated breathing system and the heat of compression that occurs when a gas cylinder is turned on too rapidly. The valve on any cylinder that contains high pressure oxygen should always be opened slowly.

On the commercial side, oxygen fires have taken place in decompression chambers, and also when divers have transferred oxygen from cylinder to cylinder. Most informed commercial diving companies prohibit their employees from transferring oxygen offshore, due to the high potential for fire and the dangers that exist when a fire occurs at sea. Of course, despite the fact that companies prohibit this practice, divers do what they feel is necessary to get the job done. One particularly bad accident took place when a diver was standing over an oxygen hose that was lying on deck. The fire started to burn inside the hose, the hose ruptured, and the lower half of the diver's body was burned.

One of the more common procedures in the commercial diving industry is called "surface-decompression on oxygen" or abbreviated as "Sur-D-O2." This practice involves having a diver complete a portion of his decompression in the water, usually at 40 FSW, and then bringing the diver to the surface where he is stripped of most of his gear, placed in a decompression chamber, and recompressed to 40 FSW to complete the balance of his decompression breathing pure oxygen in the chamber.

In the past, it was not uncommon for commercial divers to take a burning cigarette into the outer lock of the chamber as they removed the balance of their gear, before moving into the inner lock to resume oxygen breathing. One serious fire occurred on the west coast of the U.S. when a diver entered a chamber that was not ventilated properly and that contained a high percentage of oxygen. The diver was badly burned to the extent that he had almost no external ear structures left. With the decrease in smoking and better oxygen systems in chambers today, this type of accident has become much less common.

Compressor-Fill Station Accidents

While rare, compressor and fill station accidents are usually disastrous when they occur. Compressor accidents are much less common than fill station accidents, but they can and do occur.

Compressor accidents may involve belts and or plumbing that fails due to improper assembly, maintenance, or use. In these incidents, personnel or bystanders may be struck by flying debris. How-

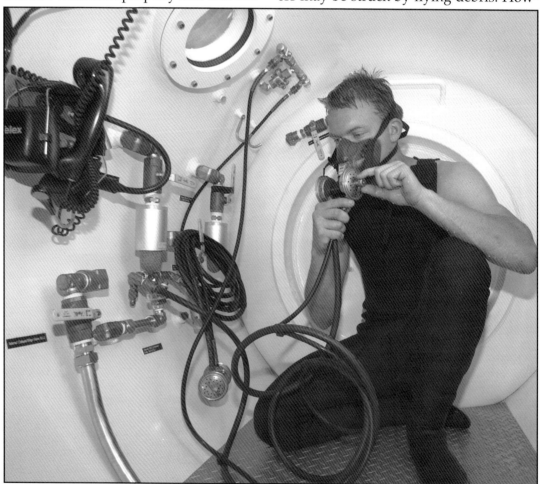

Fig. 10.1 Devastating fires have taken place inside decompression chambers when commercial divers have taken lit cigarettes into them.

ever, in most cases, belt guards and other safety equipment help to prevent this type of incident.

Fill-station accidents typically involve high-pressure cylinders that fail while they are being filled. These types of accidents are most common in the sport diving retail environment, but some commercial diving firms have high-pressure compressors that are used to fill bail-out bottles or other equipment.

High-pressure cylinders usually fail due to corrosion of the cylinder walls, but there have also been failures of aluminum cylinders that were of defective design or improperly handled. Although most cylinders are inspected on an annual basis and hydrostatically tested every five years, cylinders that have been improperly cared for can develop flaws in an extremely short period of time, particularly if they are filled with oxygen enriched gas mixtures.

Another major problem is that many fill stations are not designed according to OSHA standards, exposing both the operator and by-standers to the potential for serious injury.

When a cylinder ruptures, the force of the explosion is tremendous. These explosions can cause death or serious injury.

Eye Injuries

Over the years, eye injuries have occurred as a result of impact with various pieces of equipment. Injuries have been caused by mask lenses that have shattered, spearguns that have accidentally (or intentionally) discharged, and rup-

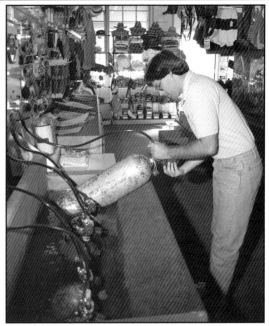

Fig. 10.2 Air station accidents may result when a cylinder fails while being filled.

tured hoses and fittings.

Although most diving equipment manufacturers now use tempered glass for scuba masks today, inexpensive masks still exist that use glass that can shatter and break into dangerous shards. In the past, these low quality masks caused devastating injuries. Today it's rare for this type of injury to occur.

Spearguns must never be cocked and loaded out of the water, but at times people make mistakes and perform this type of action. While spearguns can be lethal weapons, they have also caused less serious injuries in dive stores and other locations when they have discharged. In one case, a loaded speargun accidentally fired and the spear struck a person's eyeglasses

---

Risk Recognition for Divers and Diving Professionals

As a professional in the diving business you will undoubtedly acquire a number of different certifications and complete an extensive amount of training. In some cases, these certificates will not expire, unless you become inactive in your profession. However, most certifications will require some type of annual re-training or continuing education to maintain your proficiency. Your insurance will normally be tied to these certifications.

It's crucial that you do not let your certifications or insurance lapse for even a few days. It's important to maintain your professional status at all times.

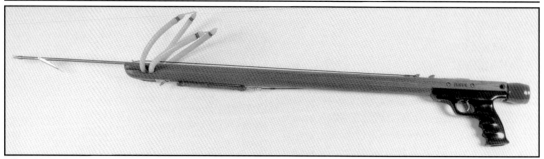

Fig. 10.3 Spearguns can cause a variety of injuries, some of which may be fatal, both in and out of the water.

causing the glass to enter the individual's eye.

Both high-pressure and low-pressure hoses on regulators and other equipment become fatigued with age and can fail. When this happens in an air environment, the hose may whip about violently. Pieces of hoses and fittings can be thrown about causing injury.

If a low-pressure hose is accidentally connected to a high-pressure orifice the hose will usually rupture, possibly sending bits of hose and/or fittings flying through the air at high speed. While most diving regulators now use different size orifices with different threads for high and low pressure fittings, older regulators did not. It's also possible to use an adapter with a newer regulator which could cause this type of incident. Serious eye injuries can occur in these situations.

Sexual Harassment

In sport diving, it's common for students to look up to their instructors with great respect. It's also not unusual for students of the opposite sex to develop crushes on their instructors.

Most recreational diving instructors are intelligent enough to realize that romantic involvements with students are best left until the course is completely over and the student has graduated. However, some instructors may "pursue" students for romantic or social purposes prior to the completion of the course. If the student has not indicated an interest in the instructor, this may be interpreted as sexual harassment.

Of course, there have also been cases where the student has been sexually attracted to the instructor and the instructor has rebuffed the student. In these circumstances, students have sometimes filed charges of sexual harassment out of embarrassment or anger.

If you are assigned to investigate a case like this for insurance purposes you must be extremely cautious in your investigation, but at the same time, very direct. Do not be afraid to ask the instructor direct questions such as:

• Did you make comments that might be considered offensive or sexually suggestive?
• Did you make sexual advances towards this student?
• Did you have, or are you having, sexual relations with this student?
• Did you make physical contact with this student in any way that might be deemed offensive?
• Did you suggest that the student's certification might be withheld if they did not submit to your sexual advances?

Slips and Falls

Given that divers are constantly climbing in and out of the water over wet rocks, entering the sea through surf, or climbing on ladders on moving boats, it's not uncommon for divers to suffer slips and falls. While the injuries from these types of accidents are rarely fatal, they can be painful and sometimes lead to disabilities.

One of the most serious slips investigated by one of the authors took place aboard a dive boat in the tropics. The boat had no guard rail or safety chain at the dive "doors" located midway along either side of the ships hull. A diver who was aboard the boat slipped on the deck, went through the open "doorway," passed under the ship and was struck by the prop, killing her instantly.

Equipment sometimes slips off a diver's body and can injure the diver who was wearing it or other individuals who happen to be standing close by. There have been several incidents where tanks have fallen out of backpacks and hit divers who were below. Weight belts sometimes slip off a diver's waist, frequently landing on the foot of the person who was wearing it and causing broken bones.

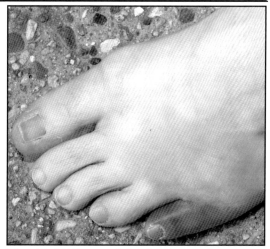

Fig. 10.4 When weights land on a diver's toes they can easily break them.

Case History – Recreational Diving

A woman in her mid-20s signed up for a diving class through a popular Florida dive store that had a good reputation for running well-taught courses and providing superior customer service. The store employed a group of instructors who were all dynamic and highly professional.

During the course, the young woman flirted with the instructor continuously. She became upset when the instructor brushed off her advances, but then (he) showed thinly disguised interest in another more mature and attractive female in the course.

On one of the ocean dives, the younger woman contended that the instructor was not in close enough proximity to her during an open water exercise to assist her when she began to experience difficulty and panicked. The instructor maintained otherwise. The woman who experienced the difficulty filed a complaint with the instructional agency and threatened a lawsuit, alleging that the instructor made sexual advances towards her.

Upon investigation of the case, it was determined that 1) the younger woman had made sexual advances towards the instructor (not the other way around), 2) the instructor was dating the more attractive woman (which he had previously denied), and 3) the instructor had <u>not</u> properly controlled the open water dive.

The facts of the case only came out after conducting interviews with every available student. This case is a good example of the necessity to interview as many people as possible who might have information that will assist you in determining the facts of the case.

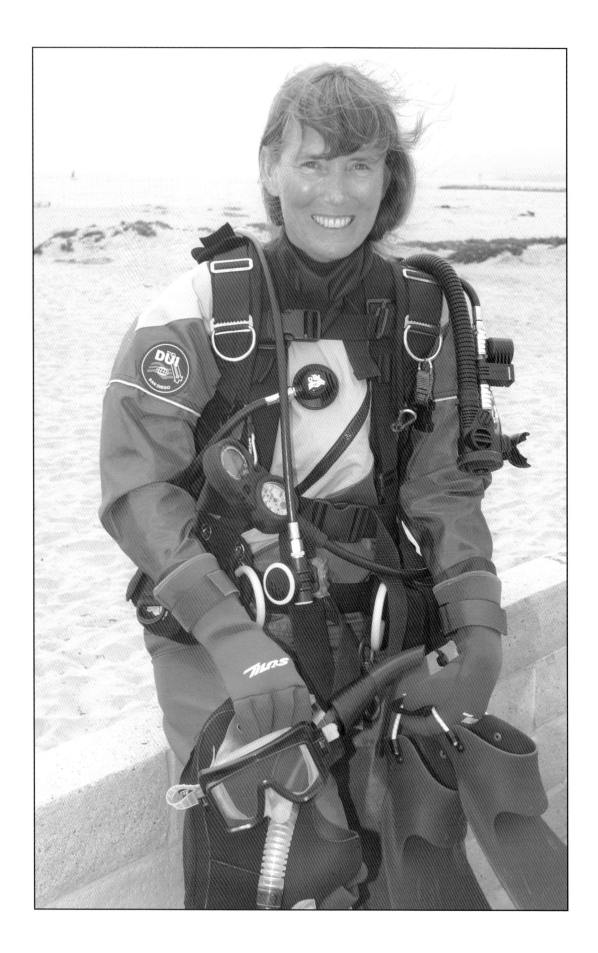

Chapter 11
What to Look for in a
Recreational Diving Accident

Investigating a recreational diving accident is quite different from investigating a commercial diving accident.

Inspecting Equipment

Any examination of diving equipment begins with the location of the equipment at the time of your examination. If you are fortunate enough to arrive on the scene of the accident itself, and the gear has been sequestered by a reliable person, there's a chance that the configuration of the gear has not been altered significantly from the way it was when it was on the victim's body. However, in almost all instances the very act of removing the equipment from the victim may have damaged the gear, or altered it from the way it was attached when it was worn.

In many cases, you may not get to examine the gear until long after the accident has taken place. During this time, the gear may have been handled by unknown persons, or stored in a location that is not conducive to maintaining the equipment in good condition. This is especially true if the equipment was stored wet in a hot, humid climate.

You are an Investigator,
Not a Tester

It is important to remember that in most cases, your examination of the gear will involve very little actual "testing," unless you have been hired as an expert witness and have been specifically assigned to test the equipment. This is an important distinction to remember because if you "test" equipment in any way that could conceivably alter its performance, you could place yourself in a challenging legal position.

It's difficult to give you an exact set of rules for what you should and should not do as an investigator, but the following are some general guidelines:

• If the scuba system is assembled and the system has not been turned off, do not turn off the air or disconnect the regulator. Mark the position of the valve handle using an indelible black marker to establish an index mark on the valve body or cylinder. Use another marker or tape to establish an index mark on the valve knob (most valve knobs are black). Count the number of turns required to close the cylinder valve and then return the valve to the position it was in.

• If the system has been disassembled, it's usually acceptable to hook the regulator up to another cylinder and briefly check the operation of the regulator, buoyancy compensator, and submersible pressure gauge on dry land.

• To check the pressure in the cylinder, we recommend the use of a stand-alone pressure gauge. This device will use the least amount of air from the cylinder, and will frequently provide a more accurate measurement than a submersible pressure gauge that may have been damaged

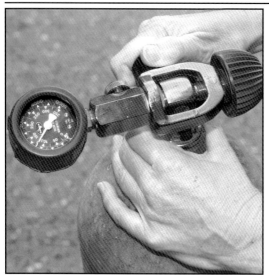

Fig. 11.1 It's best to check the pressure in the tank with a separate tank pressure gauge. If you use the victim's regulator and it free-flows you may lose a significant amount of air.

at the end of a high-pressure hose.

• If you suspect there is a possibility that the victim was using a gas mixture other than normal air; you should check the breathing gas in the cylinder to determine the percentage of oxygen in the breathing mix. You will need an oxygen analyzer to perform this check. If properly conducted, this examination uses only a miniscule amount of gas.

Keep in mind that the oxygen analyzer will only tell you how much oxygen is in the gas mixture in the cylinder, but give you no indication of what the other gas (or gases) in the tank may be. If you suspect that the gas mixture may have contributed to the accident, a laboratory will need to analyze the gas to determine whether the inert portion is helium, nitrogen, or some mixture of the two. If the cylinder must go to a laboratory for testing, be sure that you maintain a record of the chain of custody, so that you can establish who held the equipment during any given time.

Testing Equipment

In certain circumstances, you may be called upon to test the equipment in question. If this is a civil case, this will usually be done in the presence of the opposing party.

Even if you are not functioning as an expert witness, but purely as an investigator, there may be an opposing expert or investigator present when you conduct this inspection or test. Normally, there will be attorneys representing each side of the case on hand for this examination.

Before the testing is conducted, you should have a detailed discussion with the attorney for whom you are working to explain to them what you plan to do. In most cases, even attorneys who dive will not know as much about the equipment as you do, but they will usually grasp your plan readily. You should prepare a written protocol that is agreed upon by both parties in advance. You may find that you need to deviate from the protocol, but you should have a logical plan prepared before you begin. This will not only help to save time, but will usually prevent changes to the gear that may alter the results.

Be friendly but cautious in your dealings with the opposing expert or investigator. Due to the small size of the diving industry, in many cases the opposing expert will be someone who you know or who you know by reputation. Make sure that they understand and agree with the protocol you plan to follow before you begin your tests. Usually only one person will have his hands on the gear while the other person observes the exam.

Frequently, equipment testing will be videotaped for use in court. It is essential to dress appropriately and to be circumspect about your behavior and language while you are on camera.

If the inspection will be recorded on video, be sure you are aware who is paying for the recording of the video. The party paying for the video has control of the videographer and his actions. This is important because there may be times during the inspection that you want to stop recording the inspection. This should be discussed in advance with both the videographer and the attorney for whom you are working.

In a certain respect, you will be the director of the video, since the videographer will probably not know what he is looking at while he is taping. For this reason, if there is something that you think is important, it's up to you to ensure he zooms in to capture any small details that may be difficult to see.

If you can see in advance that there may be a problem with a piece of gear, or that there is the potential that a piece of gear may be damaged as a result of your action, stop the video recording, go "off the record" and discuss the problem with the attorney for whom you are working before you proceed any further. It's almost a certainty that the opposing attorney will object if this occurs, but you must not argue with them. Allow the attorneys to work this out and stay out of the debate.

Confirm Serial Numbers

The first thing to be done when you examine any equipment is to confirm the serial numbers to ensure that you are examining the correct gear. Check the serial numbers against any rental records, owner's records, or chain of custody documents. This will prevent you from wasting time by examining gear that might be from another incident, and enable you to testify with confidence should the incident end up in court. Be sure to record the location of the serial numbers on the equipment and photograph them if at all possible.

Locating the serial numbers on some equipment may be difficult, since each manufacturer marks their gear in different locations. Serial numbers may be underneath a mouthpiece on a regulator,

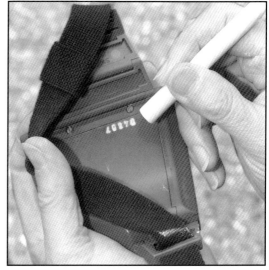

Fig. 11.2 Locating and reading the serial numbers of diving equipment can take time.

or on the back of a dive computer covered by a difficult-to-remove protective rubber shroud. If you are sure there is a serial number and it is not easily accessible, check with any attorneys who may end up handling the case before you remove a mouthpiece or do anything else that may alter the gear.

Some serial numbers are so small that they may be extremely difficult to read, or photograph, especially if they are stamped in black plastic. In this situation some white chalk can be rubbed into the engraved numbers and will help to make them easily readable.

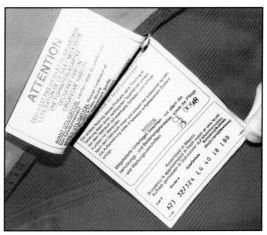

Fig. 11.3 Some buoyancy compensators may have a tag that only identifies the lot number. This may sometimes be found inside a pocket.

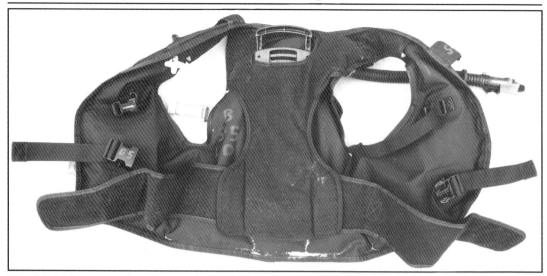

Fig. 11.4 Most rental equipment is marked with some type of identification number. Note the numbers on this buoyancy compensator, located below the right arm opening.

Serial numbers on items such as buoyancy compensators are sometimes placed inside a pocket. Some manufacturers do not serialize these items but do stamp them with a lot number.

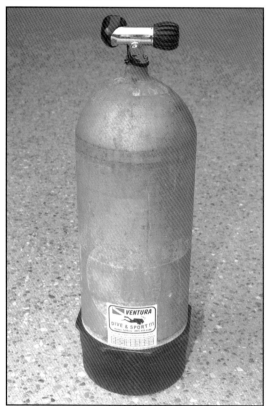

Fig. 11.5 Look for inspection or service tags on tanks and regulators. These will normally be dated and identify who performed the service.

Serial numbers on items such as fiberglass diving helmets may be cast into the helmet shell or laminated into the material.

Check Rental Numbers on Sport Scuba Gear

Many people do not own all of their own diving equipment and much of the gear involved in sport diving accidents is rental gear. In some cases, the rental markings will be obvious, but some stores are subtle about marking this property. In most cases, rental markings are crudely done by hand and will be apparent.

If the equipment is obviously rental gear the maintenance records on the equipment should be confirmed with the dive store that provided it.

Check Inspection Tags

Some facilities that perform repairs and maintenance on dive gear will routinely attach a maintenance tag to the gear when they have completed their work. When these types of tags are present there will usually be detailed information on the most recent service on the items to which they are attached.

Look for Gross Damage

Most diving equipment is extremely rugged and reliable but there are times when the equipment can be a contributory factor in accident. Any diving gear can be damaged due to neglect, impact with rocks or boats, or other unusual circumstances. Normal wear and tear is expected and should not cause the experienced investigator any undue alarm.

Certain types of wear are commonly seen, and if unchecked can lead to more serious equipment problems. For example, novice divers tend to clench regulator mouthpieces in their teeth more tightly than is necessary, and it's not unusual to see bite lugs on rental regulators that are nearly cut all the way through.

Gear that has been heavily used will have worn straps and the finish on chromed parts may be worn to the point where the underlying brass can be seen. The gear may be in perfectly functional condition although it may not be cosmetically attractive.

The types of damage that are visible to the naked eye that should provide a cause for alarm include:

- Bent or damaged valves that do not function properly
- Crushed or cracked mechanisms
- Punctures in dry suits or buoyancy compensators
- Broken zippers in dry suits

Of course, not all "damage" is visible or apparent, and a closer inspection or testing may be necessary to reveal hidden problems. For example, a commercial diver may have refinished his fiberglass helmet that was previously damaged. Also, while gear may not be technically damaged as such, its performance may be beyond the range of what is considered acceptable. This is most common with regulators, but can also occur with dive computers, tank valves, and other items.

Some of the damage that you may observe in equipment may not have taken place as part of the accident and may be entirely unrelated to the underlying cause of the accident. In addition, damage may also occur during the rescue or recovery of the victim that is also unrelated to the accident itself.

Check BC Pockets and Gear Bags

Be sure to take the time to carefully inspect the pockets of the buoyancy compensator, gear bag, and any other items that have pockets. It's possible you may find anything in these locations, including slates with handwritten notes, drugs, or other unusual items.

Anything you discover in these locations should be carefully removed, photographed, and returned to its original position.

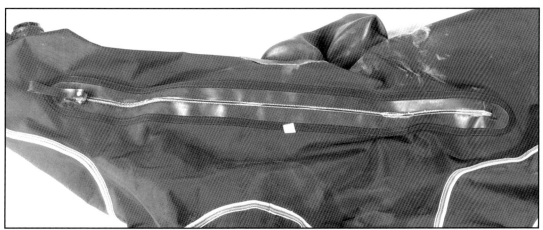

Fig. 11.6 Dry suit zippers can be broken if they are abused. This zipper had a serious leak.

Specific Inspection Points for Scuba Equipment

Mask
• Examine the skirt and strap of the mask. There should be no tears.
• Look for the presence of blood, vomitus, sand or other foreign matter in the mask. Wear gloves for your own protection.
• Note the model number/name, color, and manufacturer.

Snorkel
• Is the snorkel attached to the mask on the correct side?
• Is the mouthpiece intact?
• Note the model number/name, color, and manufacturer.

Fins
• Is the foot pocket or strap intact?
• Note the model number/name, color, and manufacturer.

Dry Suit
• Check the number of turns from fully open to fully closed for the exhaust valve. The operation of the valve should be smooth.
• Check to see if the inflator button moves freely.
• Examine the zipper carefully. There should be no missing teeth or torn base tape between the teeth. The slider should move smoothly.
• Inspect the seals and body of the suit for tears or punctures.
• Measure the circumference of the neck and wrist seal.
• Upon approval from any attorney who may be overseeing the case, seal the neck and wrist seals with rubber bands, close the exhaust valve, and inflate the suit fully to see if it holds air properly and that the valves function properly.
• Turn the dry suit inside out and inspect it carefully for the presence of stool or urine in the suit. Wear gloves for your own protection.
• Determine whether the suit was rinsed out after the accident because of the above.
• Note the manufacturer, serial number (if so marked), size, color, material, and style.

Buoyancy Compensator
• Examine all of the straps and buckles to be sure they operate correctly.
• Scrutinize the corrugated hose and check for cracks or damage that would prevent it from holding air.
• Inspect the inflator mechanism for any evidence of damage. Note the serial number of the inflator.
• Look for a label that identifies the lift capacity of the unit.
• Determine if the cylinder strap has been properly threaded.
• Check any weight pockets, especially if it is a weight-integrated BC to determine how much weight is in the buoyancy compensator.
• If the buoyancy compensator is weight integrated, upon approval from any attorney who may be overseeing the case, test the weight release mechanism for correct operation.
• Upon approval from any attorney who may be overseeing the case, inflate the BC to ensure that it holds air properly, and that the over-pressure relief valve vents air as it was designed to do.
• Note the manufacturer, serial number (if so marked), size, color, material, and style.

Cylinder Inspection
• What is the serial number of the tank?
• When was the tank manufactured?
• What color is the tank?
• What is the history of hydrostatic testing on the tank?
• When was the last time the cylinder

interior was visually inspected?

• Are there any other markings on the tank?

• Does the tank have a boot?

Cylinder Valve Inspection

• Who manufactured the valve?

• What is the condition of the o-ring?

• What is the general condition of the valve?

• How many turns does it take to turn the valve from fully closed to fully open?

• Are there any other markings on the valve?

Regulator Inspection

• Inspect for any evidence of rust on the high-pressure filter on the regulator first stage. Note the condition of the finish on the first stage.

• Confirm the presence, or absence, of a dust cap for the first stage.

• Check for loose or frozen needles in analog gauges, such as the submersible pressure gauge or depth gauge.

• If there is an analog depth gauge, see if there is a maximum depth indicating needle and note the depth that it registers.

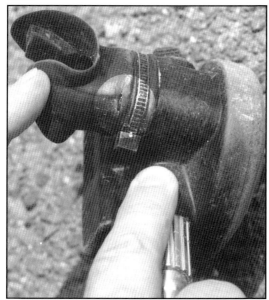

Fig. 11.7 A tear like this in a mouthpiece would let water into the regulator.

• If the instruments are in a console or rubber boot, the serial numbers are usually located under the boot.

• Record the geometry and relationship of the hoses connected to the first stage. Note any damage to the hoses.

• Examine any attached inflator hoses and see if the connecting sleeves that are used to connect them to the inflator valves slide freely.

• Look at the regulator mouthpiece and make sure it is not torn and that the lugs on the mouthpiece are present.

• Check for obviously visible foreign material (especially vomitus) in the regulator.

• If the regulator has an adjustable second stage, carefully turn the adjustment knob and see if it rotates freely. If the knob does not move easily, do not turn it any further. Note the number of revolutions from fully open to fully closed.

• Upon approval from any attorney who may be overseeing the case, connect the regulator to another tank (not the tank involved in the incident) and carefully check the normal operation of the regulator. Make a subjective note of its ease of breathing and watch for any sign of free-flow by the regulator.

• Look for any obvious cracks or damage to the second stage.

• Record the manufacturer, serial number (if so marked), color, and model. Regulators may be marked with a serial number on either the first or second stage, or both.

Regulator Testing

It is rare that the performance testing of a scuba regulator is conducted as part of a diving accident investigation. While there are many dive stores that will have a magnehelic gauge for testing the "cracking pressure" at which the second stage of a regulator flows air, there are only a small number of facilities that have "breathing machines" that can test the performance of a regulator at a simulated depth.

Deputies from the Emergency Services Detail of the Los Angeles County Sheriff's Department have routinely investigated all scuba fatalities that have occurred in the county since the 1960s. Their investigations have normally incorporated equipment testing performed at the University of California at Los Angeles, which have included regulator performance tests.

While it would be unusual for a diving accident investigator to need to conduct this type of testing, this type of examination might be included during the discovery portion of a lawsuit where equipment failure is thought to be a factor in the case.

Weight Belt

• Determine the amount of weight on the belt and the type of weights used.

• Test the operation of the quick release buckle.

• Make a note of any accessory items (knives, clips, etc.) mounted on the weight belt.

Dive Computer

Given the wide variety of dive computers on the market, it's almost impossible for anyone to understand the operation of every computer available. For this reason, you should determine the model of the computer the victim was using and obtain a manual so you know how you can access any information stored in it.

• Boot up the dive computer and verify that it completes its diagnostics properly. Make sure that there is sufficient battery power before you proceed with any further examination.

• Use the computer's log function to observe and record any dives that fall within the sequence of dives leading up to and including the accident dive itself. If the computer was owned by the victim, record the details of as many prior dives as possible.

• If the computer's data can be downloaded to a PC, download any dive data that is present and print it out as soon as possible. Have another person witness the download for authentication if at all possible.

• Be sure the dive profile downloaded from the computer matches the alleged accident dive. It is not unheard of for a computer to be hung over the side of a boat on a line in an attempt to erase old data or to support a fraudulent claim.

• Note the remaining battery power in the computer's battery and bring it to the attention of the attorneys who are managing the case if the batteries are low. Some dive computers have volatile memories and any stored data may be lost once the batteries die or are removed.

• Write down the serial number of the computer, as well as the model number, software version, and any other identifying information.

Seizing Evidence

If you are in law enforcement or are conducting an inspection on behalf of an insurance company, you may take possession of any diving equipment that was used by the accident victim, particularly in cases that resulted in serious injury or death. Of course, the ideal time to collect the gear is immediately after the accident occurs, but this is rarely possible. In most cases, several people will have handled the gear by the time you get to it.

If you do take possession of equipment in a case where civil liability issues are anticipated it's essential to do at least a minimal inspection of the gear before you transport it. You should also photograph the gear prior to transporting it so that you can substantiate its condition should any questions arise about when damage occurred. This is for your own protection as much as for the benefit of the insured parties.

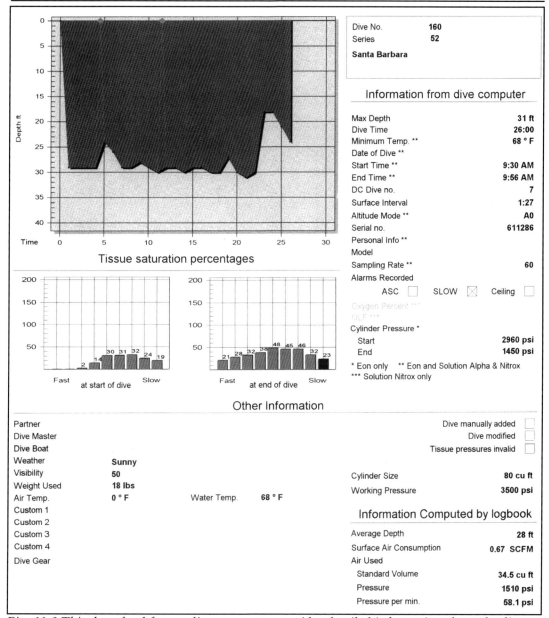

Fig. 11.8 *This download from a dive computer provides detailed information about the dive. Cables and software to obtain this information are specific to each model of computer.*

Always be sure to establish a clear chain of evidence whenever you take possession of diving equipment or deliver it to anyone else. Use signed and dated receipts each time the gear changes hands. If someone signs a receipt with an illegible scrawl, be sure to print their name next to their signature so it is clear who signed their name. It's essential to establish where the equipment has been, who handled it, and everyone who had access to it. You can't be too compulsive about this procedure.

If you are investigating on behalf of an insurance company, never put yourself in a position where you must store equipment for any length of time. As soon as possible, the gear should be delivered to the attorneys who are handling the case so that you cannot be held responsible for any loss or damage.

If you are unable to transport the equipment yourself, you must package the equipment as carefully as possible prior to shipment. Always use a premium private carrier for shipment, such as Federal Express or UPS, that provides reliable tracking.

Spoliation of Evidence

Whenever you are handling equipment that has been in a diving accident ensure that you do not alter the gear in any way. If you do accidentally damage something, you could be responsible for "spoliation of evidence," and be sued.

If you need to examine something during the course of your inspection that you think may be important and realize this could cause some change to the gear, check with the attorney to whom you are reporting and get his permission before proceeding any further. A common situation that might arise is the need to identify a serial number that is located under a regulator mouthpiece. Since certain dive equipment manufacturers stamp their serial numbers in the second stage mouthpiece tube on some regulators, the only way to read the number may be to cut the cable tie that holds the mouthpiece in

place. Before taking any action like this, be sure to get permission from whomever is supervising your investigation.

Photographing Equipment

Take several photographs of each item of equipment so that it can be positively identified. For example, if you are photographing a scuba tank, you need to start with a wide angle shot of the front and back of the tank. Take close-up shots of the tank valve, the serial numbers on the tank, any identifying rental markings, and the VIP (internal inspection) stickers.

Similarly, if you are photographing a regulator, take pictures of the complete regulator, followed by close-up pictures of the first stage, sintered bronze filter, second stage, mouthpiece, and serial numbers. All close-up shots that you take should fill the frame with the subject.

When you shoot pictures of pieces of equipment, place them against a contrasting (but neutral) background. For example, if you are photographing a black second stage regulator, don't photograph it against a dark brown carpet. Place it on

---

Risk Recognition for Divers and Diving Professionals

Every trade has its own set of standards that all individuals who are in that profession are expected to follow. This is true in both recreational and commercial diving.

In recreational diving, each individual training agency has its own set of standards. Although the standards are similar for all of the agencies, there are differences and you are expected to be familiar with your own agency's guidelines. Although you may be certified through multiple agencies, you must follow the standards required by the agency through whom you are issuing your students' certifications. If you are issuing multiple cards, you must also ensure that you meet the standards for each agency and that you do not violate your insurance agreement.

In commercial diving, the industry standard in the U.S.A. is the ADCI (Association of Diving Contractors International) Consensus Standards, but of course, regulations by OSHA and the U.S. Coast Guard also apply. In Great Britain, the Health and Safety Executive (HSE) fulfills a role similar to OSHA in the U.S.A. It is imperative that you be familiar with these different standards and that you follow them.

As a diving professional, it's your responsibility to keep abreast of the latest standards and changes and ensure compliance by you and your employees.

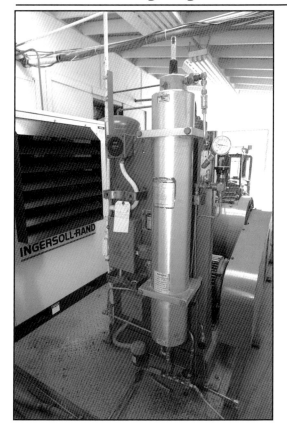

Fig. 11.9 Most dive operations are careful about keeping track of the hours and maintenance on their compressors.

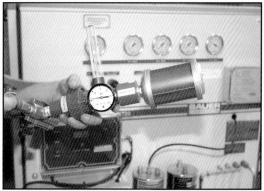

Fig. 11.10 Take an air sample from the compressor if there is any doubt about the quality of the breathing air. (Equipment courtesy of Texas Research Institute.)

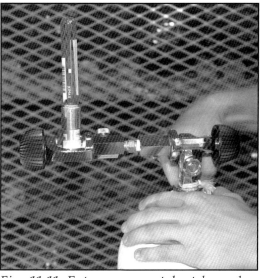

Fig. 11.11 Extra care must be taken when sampling the air from a suspect scuba cylinder that is low on air pressure.

a white towel, a sheet of light colored paper, or similar light colored background. Do not place it on a carpet with an abstract background that distracts from the subject.

Set your camera so it includes the date and time in the photograph. Also try to include a ruler in the photo so the size of the object is unambiguous.

Recreational Dive Store Records

Like all retail businesses, dive stores keep records of their personnel, their assets (such as rental gear), and other items critical to their business. These records may or may not be readily available to the investigator, depending on the type of investigation being conducted.

Rental equipment will usually have a maintenance log that at a minimum will show the last maintenance performed, who conducted it, and what parts were serviced or replaced. Obviously, serial numbers must be checked against the records to confirm the identity of the part.

Almost all dive stores regularly have the air pumped from their compressor tested by an independent laboratory. The air is analyzed for any impurities according to government standards. While it is rare for a dive store compressor to pump "bad" air, it can occur. The testing facility will normally provide the store with a certificate documenting the quality of their air.

Air Samples

As explained in the chapter on physiological factors in diving accidents, the most common contaminant in a diver's breathing air that is of concern is carbon monoxide. Although there are many laboratories that can accurately measure the level of carbon monoxide in air, even in small amounts, not all labs have the equipment needed to capture a sample of air from a scuba cylinder.

Most dive stores take air samples from their compressors on a regular basis, but not all do. Ask for a copy of the most recent air sample certificate.

Collecting air samples can be difficult, especially when you are collecting an air sample from a single scuba cylinder that is not completely full. In almost all fatal diving accidents an air sample is critical, but particularly so in a situation where the victim died for no apparent reason.

The danger in taking an air sample from a cylinder that has low pressure is that you may accidentally exhaust most of the remaining air from the cylinder. If this occurs you could be held responsible for destroying evidence.

If you must sample the air from a nearly empty scuba tank, obtain approval from the attorneys you work with prior to taking the sample. Be sure they understand the risk of losing the remaining air pressure and that they are willing to take responsibility for approving your action.

Receipts for Purchases

In a liability case, part of the paper trail that you should follow is to request all receipts that document the relationship between the person who had the diving accident and the facility providing training or rental equipment. This would include receipts for training, rentals, services (such as boat trips or equipment repairs), equipment purchases, etc. Collect every receipt, because you never know which piece of information may be crucial to the case down the road.

Training Records

In a training related accident, examine all of the documents that relate to the person's training. Generally speaking, the store or the instructor must maintain copies of each student's application for training, waiver and release, medical history, quizzes, and exams. These documents are always crucial in any case involving a student who was in training when an accident took place.

Case History – Recreational Diving

A female diver was making an advanced class dive using a dry suit in a cold water lake with poor visibility. It was the diver's third open water dive with a dry suit and the diver's training on dry suit use was incomplete.

After entering the water with her buddy, the two divers became separated. Although a search was immediately launched for the diver, she was not located until several hours later. She was found dead, on the bottom, with her weight belt in place and an empty tank, less than 200 feet from shore.

An examination of the diving equipment revealed that the waterproof zipper on the dry suit leaked badly and would not hold air. Presumably, the diver panicked and failed to drop her weight belt and/or inflate her buoyancy compensator, either of which should have allowed her to remain on the surface. Even if she had not been able to maintain positive buoyancy, she was close enough to shore to walk to shallow water on the bottom, with plenty of air left.

It's doubtful that the victim consumed all of the air in the tank. In all probability she lost control on the surface, drowned, and sank to the bottom where her regulator free-flowed and exhausted the air from the tank.

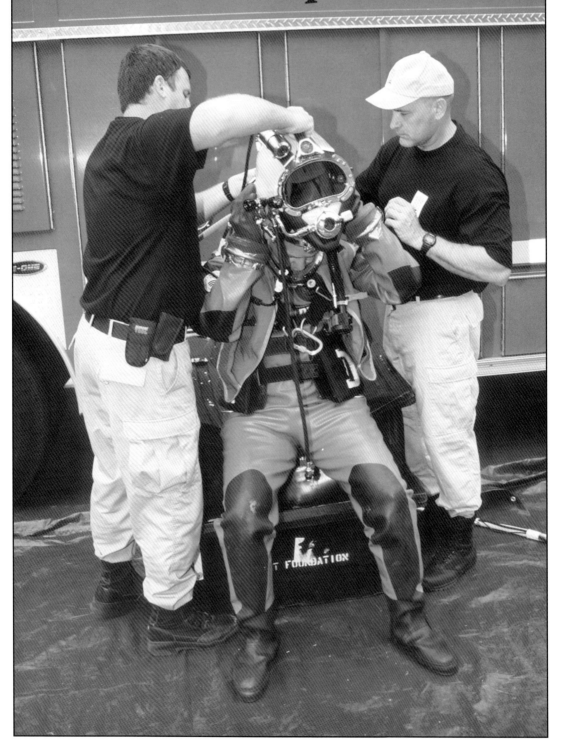

Chapter 12
Professional Diving Accidents

As mentioned previously, professional divers are generally considered to be divers who dive as part of their work, but aren't involved in the types of "heavy construction" projects performed by commercial divers. The three main types of divers who fall into this special category are scientific divers, public safety divers, and scuba instructors/dive guides.

What is a Scientific Diver?

Scientific divers are people who use diving as a tool to conduct their research. Whether they are marine biologists, archaeologists, physical oceanographers, or engaged in other types of scientific pursuits, diving is just a means for these people to get to the job site to do their work. Just as they might use a microscope to examine some interesting creature pulled up from the ocean floor, their scuba equipment is just another device for them to get the job done.

To become a scientific diver, a person must be a scientist first, and a diver second. It is apparently easier to train a scientist to be a diver than it is to train a diver to be a scientist. Similarly, in the commercial world, it may be easier to train a welder to be a diver than it is to train a diver to be a welder.

Scientific divers are required to undergo more extensive training than the average recreational scuba diver. Most scientific diving courses include a minimum of 100 hours of instruction and 12

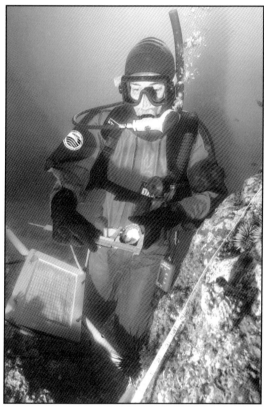

Fig. 12.1 Scientific divers primarily make observations, take measurements, and shoot photos.

open water dives. In addition, most scientific divers get additional training in specialized equipment like dry suits or surface-supplied gear.

Who Employs Scientific Divers?

Scientific divers are most commonly employed by state or federal agencies. For example, in California, the Department of Fish and Game employs marine biologists who use diving to conduct field studies on the different biological resources of the state.

At the federal level, there are numerous agencies that use diving to do their work, including organizations like the Environmental Protection Agency (EPA), the National Park Service, and the National Oceanic and Atmospheric Administration (NOAA). These organizations have divers working around the world on various projects.

Many universities, consulting firms, and marine aquariums also employ scientific divers.

Scientific Diving and the OSHA Exemption

Scientific divers have a specific exemption from the OSHA regulations that apply to commercial diving. This exemption is based upon the excellent safety record these divers have maintained.

To be eligible for the OSHA exemption, an organization that is engaged in scientific diving must have a diving safety officer and a diving control board, comprised of members of the organization who oversee the diving. In addition, there are other requirements that include:

- No construction or other heavy work may be performed.
- The organization must have a set of scientific diving regulations.
- Divers may only be certified for specific depths, for example, a newly certified scientific diver may only be authorized to dive to 33 feet or shallower. Experience must be gained under supervision before they are allowed to operate at successively deeper depths.
- The divers must adhere to the buddy system.
- Information and data resulting from the scientific project are for the advancement of science and non-proprietary.

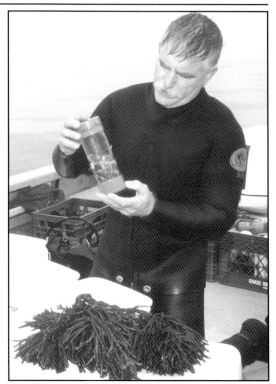

Fig. 12.2 Scientific divers are not governed by the OSHA diving regulations.

American Academy of Underwater Sciences (AAUS)

The American Academy of Underwater Sciences is the umbrella association in the United States to which most scientific divers and their organizations belong. The Academy was the outgrowth of the scientific diving community's negotiations with OSHA regarding the exemption of scientific divers from the OSHA regulations. Each year the Academy hosts a meeting of diving safety officers from various institutions across the U.S. at which current practices in scientific diving are reviewed.

In addition to the diving officers' meeting, the academy also sponsors an annual conference on scientific diving.

The Role of the Diving Safety Officer

Diving safety officers are usually full-time employees at most research facilities where scientific diving is conducted. It is the responsibility of the diving safety officer to ensure that all diving operations that are conducted under the auspices of their organization follow the diving practices set out in their respective diving manual. At a large university, the diving safety officer will usually report to the campus safety director, but also takes direction from the diving control board.

Some of the duties that fall to the diving safety officer include:

- Training new scientific divers
- Reviewing the dive logs of all divers in the program to ensure they are following proper procedures.
- Ensuring that all equipment used by divers in the program has been serviced each year.
- Performing check-out dives with divers visiting from other programs.
- Accompanying divers from the program on their operations to ensure that they are following safe practices.

Scientists Do Many Types of Work

Scientific divers do many different types of research, depending upon their area of specialization. Most of the work they do is limited to making observations and collecting specimens or artifacts.

Biologists typically will count specimens, tag animals, or observe behaviors, and other similar tasks. Archaeologists will map sites, recover artifacts, or photograph wrecks.

Scientists Use Many Types of Gear

While most diving scientists use scuba as their primary mode of diving, they may also use other equipment, including rebreathers and surface-supplied gear. They also use many types of specialized scientific devices to assist them in their work. These devices may be as simple as measuring tapes and calipers, or as sophisticated as time lapse photographic

equipment in special housings.

Scientific Diving Sites

Scientists dive in many different types of environments, some of which are quite unusual and outside the realm of normal recreational diving. For example, while some sport divers participate in ice diving, few enter environments that are as hostile as the Antarctic, where scientists regularly dive. There has been at least one scientific diving fatality in this part of the world, with a researcher who was inadequately trained in dry suit diving techniques.

Another unusual environment where scientists conduct biological research is in the open ocean, where scientists who dive here use a special arrangement known as a "trapeze" to control their depth and provide them with an orientation to the surface. This type of open ocean diving is more commonly referred to as "bluewater diving," where the bottom of the ocean may be thousands of feet below the diver. One of the common tasks for divers in these environments is to collect free floating plankton specimens.

The trapeze is a device designed to help provide the divers with a frame of reference and to help prevent the divers from accidentally descending below their maximum planned depth. Diving without a reference to the bottom and with no vertical frame of reference can be extremely disorienting. The trapeze uses a pulley and a light counterweight to help the diver maintain an orientation to the surface.

Prior to the standardization of the techniques for this type of diving, there was at least one blue water diving accident. In this case, the scientific team conducting an open ocean dive used a 50-pound weight, that one of the divers tied onto with a shorter line using a knot that could not be released. When the line carrying the weight snapped close to the surface, the diver did not have sufficient

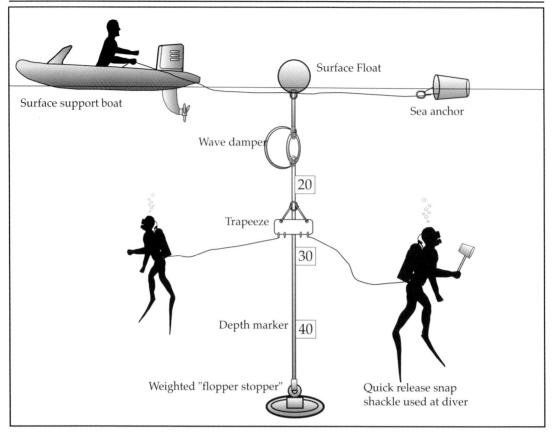

Fig. 12.3 The procedures for blue-water diving have been standardized and are widely recognized today as essential for this type of diving.

buoyancy with her BC to offset the weight to which she was attached. She was unable to release herself from the line, and was dragged to her death in thousands of feet of water. Her body was never recovered. Procedures for blue-water diving were standardized following this incident.

What is a Public Safety Diver?

Public safety divers are people who go underwater for the benefit of the population of a particular city, county, state, or the entire nation. Included in the ranks of these divers are the following:

- Firefighters
- Law enforcement personnel (police, sheriffs, FBI, game wardens, etc.)

These divers must frequently work in extremely challenging environments and under hazardous conditions. Typically, they are highly motivated but often they are inadequately equipped.

This high level of motivation combined with inadequate equipment, training, and practice creates a situation with a high number of accidents each year.

Diving is just a part of the job

For most public safety divers, diving is just a part of their job. Only in rare instances do these divers get in the water daily. For example, the divers who work for the New York Harbor Patrol are also peace officers, but their primary mission is to dive to recover evidence, retrieve bodies, and perform rescues. They are the exception rather than the rule, because most public safety divers do not dive frequently.

In many cases, the divers who staff the local search and recovery team are volunteers from the general public. This is particularly common in rural areas where the funding for this type of operation may be minimal or non-existent.

Many problems occur with volunteer dive teams due to a lack of funding. These challenges often indirectly lead to diving accidents. Some of the issues that public safety dive teams face include:

• Lack of standardization of equipment
   Many divers on volunteer teams supply their own equipment and divers may use their own personal sport diving equipment. In situations where divers are working in black water, this lack of familiarity with another team member's equipment can make it difficult for one diver to assist another who is having a problem with his equipment.

• Inadequate equipment for the dive
   Public safety divers frequently must dive in waters that are highly polluted or at deeper depths. If there is no funding for the dive team, these highly motivated individuals may try to "make do" with the equipment they have, sometimes with disastrous results.

• Inadequate training
   It's not uncommon for individuals on volunteer dive teams to receive little training beyond their recreational scuba training. When faced with a difficult situation, their training may not be up to the task at hand.

• Inadequate maintenance of training
   Diving is the type of activity that should be regularly practiced for a person to maintain both his proficiency and his comfort level in the water. The typical volunteer team does not get sufficient practice to maintain their skills.

Public Safety Divers Have An OSHA Exemption

Like scientific divers, public safety divers have a special exemption from the

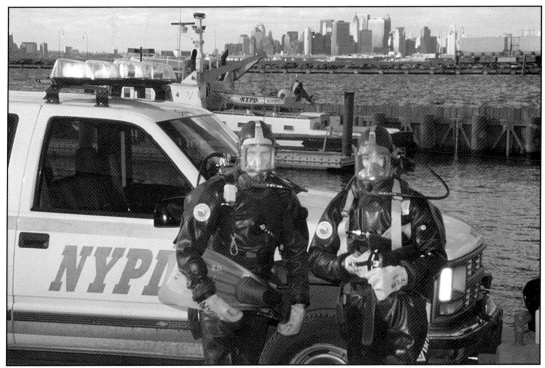

Fig. 12.4 Divers with the New York City Harbor Patrol are police officers and dive every day as part of their job. Most of their dives are made in conditions where the visibility underwater is no more than a few inches at best, but more frequently with no visibility.

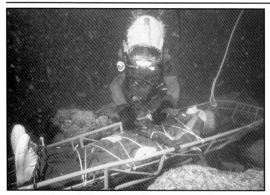

Fig. 12.5 Public safety divers must frequently dive in contaminated water. (Photo by Steve Barsky. © Kirby Morgan Dive Systems, Inc. All rights reserved.)

OSHA regulations that govern commercial diving. However, since public safety divers are usually employees, OSHA still has an interest in their welfare. Technically speaking, even a volunteer diver is considered an employee by OSHA's definition if that person receives their equipment as a "perk" for their contributions of time.

In some states, state-enforced OSHA regulations do specifically address public safety diving, but this is generally the exception rather than the rule.

Public Safety Diving Equipment

Public safety divers use much of the same equipment that is used by recreational divers, although in many cases, they should be using equipment that is more suitable for commercial diving. Since much of the diving done by these divers is conducted in harbors, drainage canals, irrigation ditches, and inner city ponds, they are frequently exposed to chemical and biological contaminants from which sport diving equipment will not protect them. In addition, they regularly dive in water that has low or zero visibility and therefore they should be outfitted with communications equipment.

The emerging basic standard for public safety divers appears to be a dry suit, full-face mask, and wireless or hard-wire communications. This is the minimum gear required to help protect divers from polluted waters and provide acceptable thermal protection in colder waters.

Public Safety Diving Standards

Unfortunately, there are no universally accepted standards for public safety diving. The National Association of Search and Rescue (NASAR) has developed a diving standard that addresses some, but not all, of the issues faced by public safety divers. Likewise, the National Fire Protection Association has developed a standard for firefighters who

---

Risk Recognition for Divers and Diving Professionals

In the U.S., there is no annual recertification requirement for recreational divers, and for most divers this is not a problem. However, each year, there are a number of accidents or near misses that involve divers who have not been diving for some time, or who get back into the water without any type of refresher course. This is a situation that has a high potential for accidents and is one that anyone who provides diving services should recognize.

In the scientific diving community, there has always been a strong requirement for a minimum number of dives that each diver must log annually. In addition, many organizations hold some type of annual recertification course and have a requirement for additional training and annual fitness tests.

The public safety diving community would do well to consider adopting training strategies similar to the scientific diving community to lower its accident rate and improve safety. This is not as much of a problem for full-time public safety dive teams as it is for some volunteer organizations.

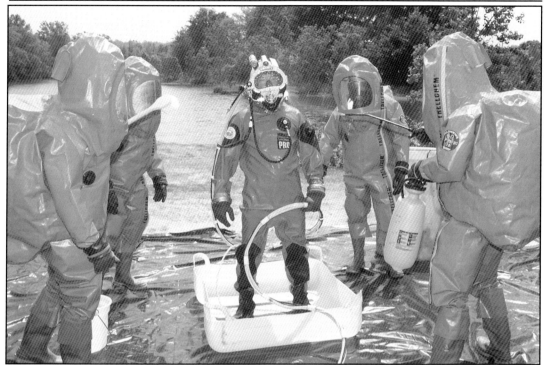

Fig. 12.6 Public safety divers frequently use much of the same gear used by commercial divers.

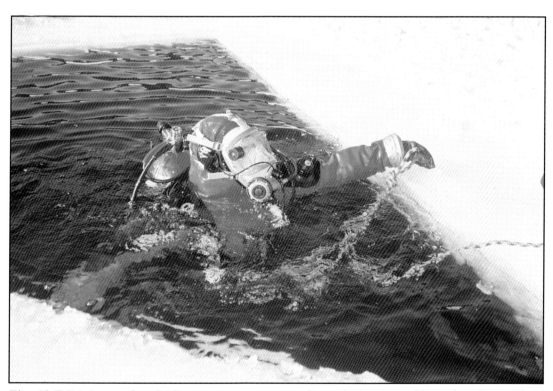

Fig. 12.7 Diving under the ice presents numerous hazards for the public safety diver. These may include regulator freeze-up, loss of the entry/exit hole, and hypothermia. (© Dave Jephson. All rights reserved.)

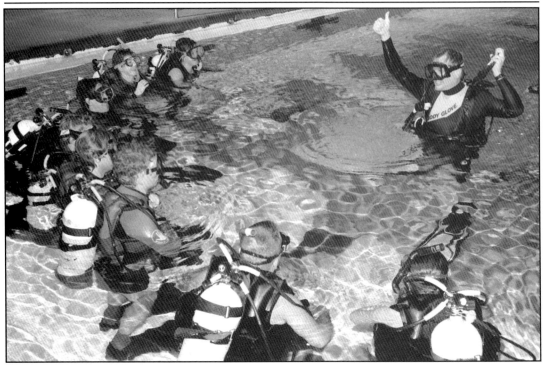

Fig. 12.8 Like scientific divers, recreational diving instructors are also exempt from the OSHA diving regulations.

dive, but their standard does not cover law enforcement personnel.

Public Safety Diving Accidents

Public safety divers work under conditions that most sport divers will never experience. Given the relatively small number of public safety divers (approximately 5,000), there are a disproportionately high number of public safety diving accidents each year. On an annual basis, there are usually about four public safety diving accidents, and about 70% of these occur during training. This is a high number of training accidents, but not surprising when you consider the limited training most of these divers received for the demanding dives they make.

Recreational Scuba Instructors

Recreational scuba instructors are another group that are not regulated by OSHA. Accidents involving instructors are rare, but occasionally they do occur. More often than not, it is the student who is hurt during training. Although this al-

most invariably leads to an investigation, the inquiry is that of the sport diving accident.

Instructors employed as dive guides tend to work long hours and may make multiple dives, many days in a row. Although it is rare to hear of an instructor death in a diving accident, decompression sickness probably occurs with fairly high regularity among diving instructors.

Since instructors tend to be more experienced divers, they frequently make dives that are more challenging and have more risk. More instructors are probably involved in diving accidents when they are not teaching, than when they have students in the water. In the Divers Alert Network (DAN) 2002 report (based on year 2000 data) on diving accidents, instructors represented approximately 10% of the population of divers suffering from decompression sickness.

While teaching, instructors must make many more ascents and descents during a day than their students. If a student panics and bolts for the surface, the instructor may be forced to make a rapid ascent in an effort to regain control of the student.

Of the 91 divers who died in 2000, two were instructors. In the general diving population there are certainly less diving instructors than other certification levels. However, instructors probably make many more dives a year than your "average" diver, so their exposure to risk is greater.

Case History – Commercial Diving

A commercial diver was working in shallow harbor water when observers noticed that he had surfaced and was "thrashing around." This activity ceased and a skiff was put into the water in an attempt to render aid. Upon arrival at the diver the rescuers found the diver to be motionless.

He was hoisted to the skiff and then to a working barge where his gear was removed and he was found to be pulseless and apneic. CPR was attempted and he was brought to a medical facility where attempts at resuscitation were unsuccessful.

He was declared dead and an autopsy was performed. The results of the autopsy confirmed that the cause of death was an air embolism (however the pathologist had to be given a copy of a protocol for victims of diving accidents as he originally thought the cause of death was drowning).

Further investigation and other aspects of the autopsy revealed multiple additional factors that raised as many questions as were answered. Most importantly, bite marks were found inside the diver's mouth on his tongue, and stool was found in his diving suit. Along with this, his gums were enlarged in a fashion caused by the drug phenytoin (an anticonvulsant drug) and another anticonvulsant drug (phenobarbital) was found in his blood stream. Finally on initial testing of the diver's blood trace amounts of cocaine were found, but this could not be reconfirmed on further testing.

There were reports that the diver was having trouble with the inflation valve on his dry suit. In this case, the thorough investigation that was performed in this fatality did not answer the ultimate question of exactly what happened to this diver. It seems clear he had a seizure, however whether this was the cause of his air embolism or the consequence of it could not be determined. The diver may have had a seizure and because of a possible "leaky" intake valve, he could have ascended while having the seizure, causing an air embolism.

Concern was also raised that the difficulty the diver was experiencing with his dry suit valve caused an uncontrolled ascent, which in turn was the cause of the AGE and the seizure was a result of the uncontrolled ascent. The exact sequence of events will never be known but certainly had the diver's employers known that the diver had an underlying seizure disorder (epilepsy) he would not have been cleared to dive. OSHA standards are clear in this respect; individuals with an underlying seizure disorder are not candidates for commercial diving.

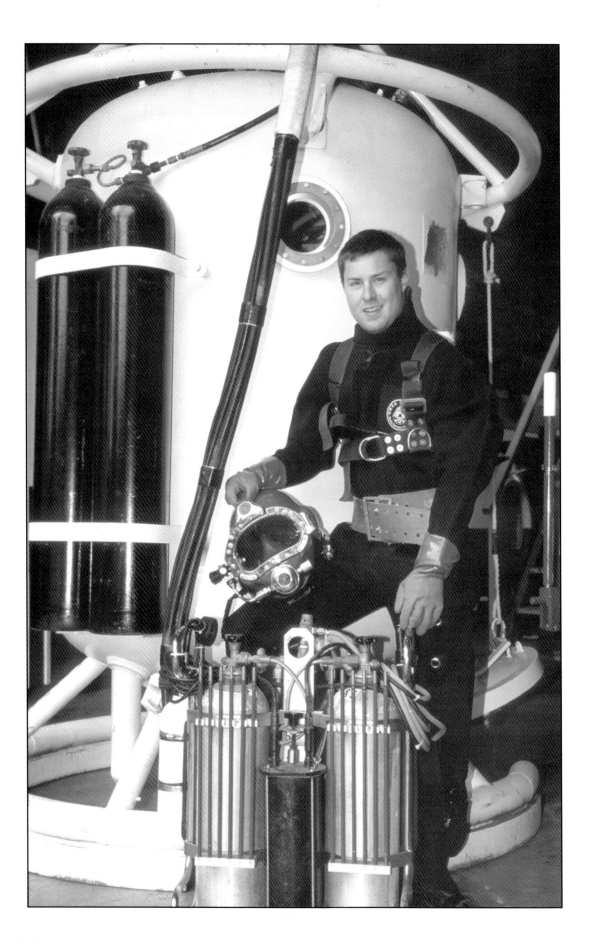

Chapter 13
Commercial Diving Accidents

Investigating a commercial diving accident is obviously quite different than investigating a sport diving accident. Not only are you dealing with an industrial environment, but you are also dealing with different equipment, different motivations, social factors, and regulations. If you do not have experience working in a construction environment, you will probably have a difficult time investigating a commercial diving accident.

During the period 1996-2000 the U.S. Coast Guard received reports on six commercial diving fatalities (excluding deaths of professional seafood divers). This does not include commercial diving deaths in waters that do not fall under the jurisdiction of the U.S.C.G.

The Organizational Environment in Commercial Diving Companies

Larger commercial diving companies have a fairly formal, organized structure that is used to assign responsibility for various aspects of their business. Smaller companies are generally more loosely organized. In order to conduct an investigation you must determine who is responsible for what aspects of the organization in order to question the appropriate people.

Bigger commercial diving companies typically work on large-scale jobs, which often include oilfield work or deepwater projects such as bridges or dams that span greater depths. It takes a big organization with lots of manpower to support a div-

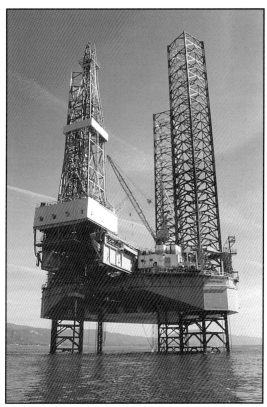

Fig. 13.1 Most oilfield diving operations are performed by the larger commercial diving companies.

ing job in 300 FSW. Smaller companies tend to work on inland and inshore projects such as docks, piers, sewer outfalls, and other jobs in less than 190 FSW.

Almost all commercial diving companies hire seasonal personnel as job demands change. It is not uncommon for a diver to move from one company to another and back again during the course of his career.

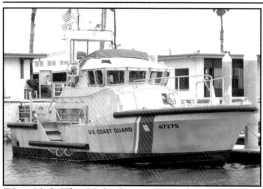

Fig. 13.2 The U.S. Coast Guard investigates diving accidents that fall under its jurisdiction in light of its regulations.

Most diving companies today are members of the Association of Diving Contractors International (ADCI). This is a trade association for the commercial diving industry that promotes safety in commercial diving operations. If a company is not a member of the ADCI, they may not be following the standards of the association.

Along the west coast of the United States, some divers belong to the Dock Workers and Pile Drivers union, which has its own set of rules for diving on the job. Divers may belong to unions in other parts of the world, too.

Commercial Diving Regulations

Aside from the industry's own standards, both the United States Coast Guard (USCG) and the Federal Occupational Safety and Health Administration (OSHA) have regulations in place that govern commercial diving operations. There is some overlap in these regulations, and some areas that neither set of regulations addresses.

While there has been continued talk about the wholesale adoption, or adaptation, of the ADCI standards by both OSHA and the U.S. Coast Guard, there is no target date set for this to occur. It seems doubtful that it will occur in the near future.

In most civil lawsuits, the opposing parties will closely scrutinize the OSHA and USCG regulations to see which parts, if any, are applicable and if the diving company has violated any part of these standards. Since most attorneys are not familiar with these regulations, or the issues raised in them, they will usually rely on their investigators and/or experts to help them interpret the accident in light of these regulations and standards.

OSHA Diving Regulations

The OSHA Commercial Diving Standards have been published as part of the Federal Register, Part 1910 - Occupational Safety and Health Standards, Subpart T-Commercial Diving Operations. This document is available in its entirety on the Internet.

The OSHA regulations apply to anyone who is working as a diver within the waters of the U.S. and its territories or within the Outer Continental Shelf. The region of the Outer Continental Shelf is defined in another Federal document, 67 Stat. 462, 43 U.S.C. 1331.

OSHA diving regulations do **not** apply to people who are teaching recreational sport diving, performing search and rescue operations for a governmental agency, or are performing scientific research under an organized scientific diving program. These groups are exempt from following the OSHA standards, although there are standards that are applicable to each of these environments.

The regulations are applicable to situations where there is an employer/employee relationship. A self-employed seafood diver working from a small boat, is not subject to the OSHA regulations.

The regulations address many issues including personnel requirements, procedures, diving equipment, and record keeping. Most diving contractors who are members of the ADCI are well aware of the OSHA diving regulations, and strive to ensure that their operations are in compliance with the law.

State Regulations

Many states have their own labor laws that serve to supplement the federal OSHA regulations. While federal laws take precedence over state laws, it's possible that the state diving regulations may address issues with which OSHA does not deal.

If the accident that you are investigating took place within state waters, you should determine if there are any applicable state labor laws.

In 2003, a total of 27 states are covered by Federal OSHA regulations, while 23 states have their own OSHA plans, which must meet or exceed Federal standards.

U.S. Coast Guard Diving Regulations

The U.S. Coast Guard has their own set of standards that have also been published in the Federal Register as Subchapter V – Marine Occupational Safety and Health Standards, Title 46CFR, Part 197, Subpart B – Commercial Diving Operations.

The USCG regulations govern diving operations that occur in deepwater ports, the safety zone surrounding deepwater ports, any permanent or temporary structure on the Outer Continental Shelf (such as an oil platform), and all vessels that must have a USCG certificate of inspection. The same exemptions for sport diving, public safety divers, and scientific divers that OSHA recognizes are also acknowledged by the Coast Guard.

USCG regulations do not cover commercial diving operations taking place in shallow pleasure boat harbors, landlocked lakes, shallow rivers, or similar locations, unless pollution is an issue (such as an oil or chemical spill). Under normal operations at inland (inshore) locations, the OSHA standards apply. The USCG has strict rules regarding their notification in the event of a fatality, or an event in which a person is hospitalized for more than 24 hours, or incapacitated for more than 72 hours.

During an oil spill or hazardous substance release, the National Contingency Plan, (40 CFR 300) requires that response operations, including commercial diving operations, be conducted in accordance with the requirements, standards and regulations of OSHA (29 CFR 1910).

The U.S. Coast Guard Takes Diving Accidents Seriously

The U.S. Coast Guard takes commercial diving accidents very seriously and has performed many detailed investigations.

A 1993 Coast Guard Marine Casualty report of a commercial diver killed while burning with a cutting torch underwater is a case in point. At the time of the accident, the diver was wearing a diving helmet that had been extensively modified by the user. Key suspension elements for the diver's head had been removed, the oral-nasal mask was changed, and snaps

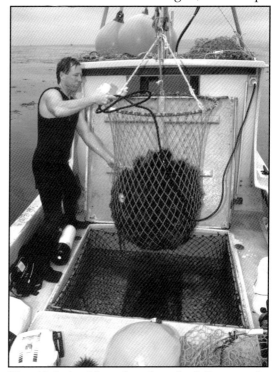

Fig. 13.3 A self-employed seafood diver working from his own boat is not subject to the OSHA commercial diving regulations. This diver is hauling in a load of sea urchins.

to accommodate another manufacturer's head cushion had been installed. In essence, the helmet had been "gutted" to allow the modifications that changed the performance of the diver's life support gear and compromised the diver's safety. The helmet consequently fitted loosely on the diver's head and most probably came off during the explosion. During the investigation, these modifications became obvious.

In another investigation, in 1997, a commercial diving company supplied copies of air sample analyses to a U.S.C.G. investigator. Upon examination, the investigator noted that something about the computer generated reports didn't look right. Additionally, the signature of the lab representative was identical on each report.

When the investigator contacted the laboratory that supposedly had conducted the analysis, he discovered that the person who had "signed" the reports had died three years earlier. Obviously, the company was falsifying their equipment maintenance records. The Coast Guard actually began a criminal investigation of the diving company and it subsequently ceased operation.

Common Sites of Commercial Diving Accidents.

Most accidents investigated by the U.S.C.G. center on the Gulf of Mexico, with investigators based out of Morgan City, Louisiana and Port Arthur, Texas. This should come as no surprise since this is the area where the bulk of the commercial diving activity in the U.S. occurs.

Diving Operations Management

The management of most larger commercial diving companies is made up of former divers, engineers, and some purely business personnel with no commercial diving background. Management usually has little direct contact with the daily operations in the field, but will usually interface with senior diving superintendents and supervisors.

Smaller diving companies, those with less than 50 total employees, will usually be less formal. Their personnel may wear many different hats and both management and field personnel may interact directly. In a very small diving company (with less than 20 personnel) an investigator may end up interviewing the president of the company, who may have been on the job in the field when the accident took place.

Operations Manager (Ops Manager)

Most larger diving companies will have an operations manager, whose job it is to oversee all of the diving operations of the company. They also make recommendations to management regarding the acquisition of equipment. It's the operation manager's job to pick the personnel and equipment for the job, to interface with the customer, and hire (and fire) divers.

The diving operations manager will be an experienced diver who no longer works in the field. Operations managers often retire from field work due to family responsibilities, injuries, age, or health issues that prevent them from actively diving. They normally do not go offshore, but oversee all of the company's jobs, hire personnel, perform personnel reviews, and give job assignments from the company office.

When a diving accident occurs, the operations manager will normally be the first person that the offshore diving supervisor will call. The operations manager will normally assist with making any arrangements for personnel evacuation or decisions regarding extended decompression treatment. If the company has an operations manager, he will usually have knowledge of whatever events took place. He should be interviewed.

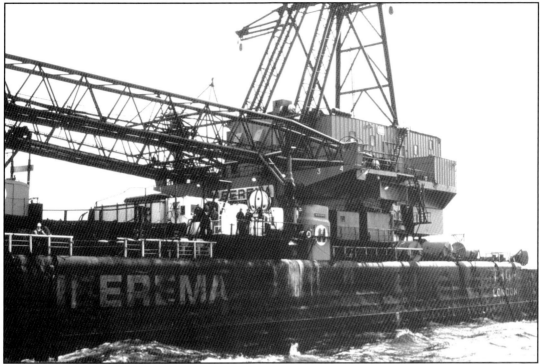

Fig. 13.4 It takes a large commercial diving company to supply the continuous manpower on a long-term major construction job.

Diving Superintendent

Big diving companies may have diving superintendents who roam from job to job offshore to ensure that the company's operations are proceeding smoothly. If a job is not moving ahead at the proper pace, the superintendent may stay on the job until any problems are solved.

It's usually quite rare for a superintendent to dive, but on occasion they may do so to personally see what issues are holding up the job.

Unless a superintendent is actually on the job site when an accident takes place, he usually will have no more knowledge of the incident than other personnel ashore.

Shift Supervisor

Most oilfield diving jobs are conducted on a 24-hour a day schedule, seven days a week. This means that the diving crew works around the clock, weather and other conditions permitting, until the job is complete. In this situation, there will be two separate crews, one working the night shift and one on the day shift. The night shift will typically run from midnight until noon and the day shift will run from noon to midnight.

The size of the crew will be contingent on the complexity and depth of the job. In most circumstances, the deeper the water, the larger the crew.

The shift supervisor must be qualified for the type of diving being conducted. Large companies typically will have three different types of diving supervisors:

• Saturation diving supervisors – qualified to run any type of diving operation, including saturation, surface-supplied mixed gas, and air diving.

• Mixed gas diving supervisor – qualified to run both mixed gas and air diving operations.

• Air diving supervisor – qualified to run only air diving operations.

The shift supervisor will usually have intimate knowledge of any incident that has taken place on the job. In most cases, he will be in direct communication with the diver in the water.

Rack Operator

On larger diving jobs, especially on operations such as mixed gas or saturation dives, there may be a person whose sole function is to run the gas mixtures and operate the communications for the diver in the water. This person is normally designated as the "rack operator," which means he is running the divers gas control manifold or "rack."

When there is a rack operator who is also handling communications, this person will be communicating with the diver rather than the shift supervisor. However, at times, the shift supervisor may take over the communications if the diver is having difficulty with the job, or the rack operator needs to be relieved to use the "head," or to get a meal.

The shift supervisor will normally be in the dive control van with the rack operator, although there may be times when he leaves the van to check on deck operations. If there is a customer's representative on the job, the shift supervisor may also be engaged in conversations with the client and may not be directly monitoring the dive. This is normal and does not in any way denote that the supervisor is not doing his job.

In some cases, the "rack operator" may actually be a diver, who is merely fulfilling the function of the job as part of the rotation of personnel on the job. Conversely, in other companies, the rack operator may have no other duties.

A good rack operator will be able to judge how comfortable the diver is underwater by listening to his breathing and his speech. He must be attuned to changes in the diver's behavior or breathing pattern and know when the diver's stress level is increasing.

On an air diving job, the rack operator's job is very straightforward. He has three main responsibilities. First, he must keep track of the diver's bottom time and decompression status. Secondly, he must monitor the diver's air supply pressure. Third, he must communicate with the diver and direct the tenders to lower tools to the diver as needed, and instruct the

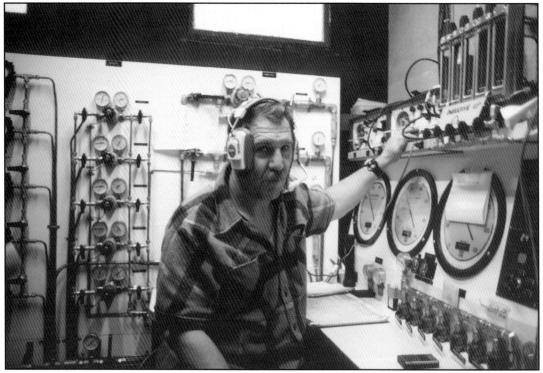

Fig. 13.5 The life support technicians maintain the log for the saturation system.

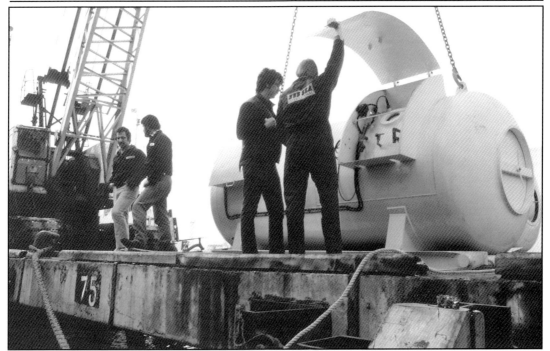

Fig. 13.6 Teamwork is essential on a commercial diving job and divers must have many skills to be considered a valuable part of the team.

deck crew to pull up on the diver's hose when needed or slack it off as he moves deeper. If the diver is using a hot water suit, the rack operator will also be responsible for controlling the temperature of the water supplied to the diver's suit.

On a mixed-gas or bell-saturation diving job, the rack operator's job becomes more complex, because there will normally be gas mixture changes as the diver travels to and from the bottom. The diver will use mixtures containing less oxygen as he moves deeper and mixtures richer in oxygen as he returns to shallower depths. The rack operator must ensure that the diver gets the proper gas mixture at the right time.

Life-Support Technician

On a saturation diving job that involves round-the-clock diving, there will usually be one man on each shift whose sole responsibility is to attend to the divers who are living in the saturation chamber complex on the deck of the ship. This person is known as the "life-support technician" or "life-support tech."

The life-support tech has many tasks to perform including the following:

• Maintaining the saturation system at the correct temperature and humidity for the comfort of the divers.

• Maintaining the proper levels of oxygen and carbon dioxide in the chamber environment.

• Locking in food and fluids to the divers.

• Keeping a log of all medical lock runs, toilet flushes, carbon dioxide absorbent changes, decompression, and other actions tending to the divers in the chamber.

Lead Diver

Lead divers are highly experienced divers who are expected to run the operations on the deck of the ship while the diving supervisor runs the diving manifold and communications to the diver. It's the lead diver's responsibility to see to it that the diver in the water gets the equipment he needs lowered to him and that the diver's hose is tended properly. The lead diver will generally be the most

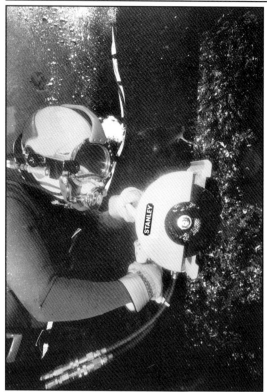

Fig. 13.7 Almost any of the tools commercial divers use can produce serious injuries if they are handled improperly. This diver is using a hydraulic saw. (Photo by Steve Barsky. © Kirby Morgan Dive Systems, Inc. All rights reserved.)

knowledgeable person on the deck.

Lead divers are normally part of the diving rotation. They are frequently assigned to the more complex or demanding dives, or to dives that pay a substantial depth premium (as a reward for their other responsibilities on deck).

Lead divers are usually being groomed to be shift supervisors, and in a large company that does mixed-gas and saturation diving, a lead diver may frequently be assigned to supervise an air diving job. Lead divers are generally expected to be thoroughly familiar with all of the deck equipment, decompression procedures, and other management aspects of the job.

Divers

As a commercial diver, a person is supposed to be a skilled underwater laborer who is capable of going underwater in demanding conditions to perform useful work. In most companies today, a diver is expected to be a "jack-of-all-trades" with a variety of skills that make him useful both topside and underwater. A diver is expected to have at least rudimentary knowledge of plumbing, welding, engine and compressor maintenance, small-boat handling skills, mechanical drawing, technical report writing, as well as other talents.

In most countries in the world today, you cannot become a commercial diver without having first graduated from an accredited commercial diving school. This training is really only the first step towards becoming a diver, because most companies do not hire diving school graduates as divers but as apprentices or "tenders" as described below. It takes time for most tenders to gain the on-the-job experience needed to actually become a diver.

A person who has just been promoted to the position of "diver" in a company is generally referred to as a "break-out diver." New divers, unless they are extremely talented, are usually not assigned to the more demanding or higher paying jobs, unless the diver has specific talents that are needed on a particular job.

To be a good diver, a person must have a "can-do" attitude, that translates into confidence and a determination to get the job done. Yet, being a good diver does not mean placing yourself at risk, and the smart diver usually knows when the risks on a job are too high.

A diver always has the right to decline to dive, and a good diver will know when the situation presents hazards that are unacceptable. However, group psychology may cause people to refrain from voicing their concerns for fear of looking foolish or being branded as a coward.

Diving jobs that were operating at a cost of tens of thousands of dollars a day have been shut down by divers when the perils of the job appeared to be too great. In a positive job environment, the dive team will normally be supportive once one of its members identifies an unacceptable threat to safety.

Most divers will readily admit that they have had times when they have been scared underwater, either because something went wrong on the job, or the work was different from how they perceived it would be prior to the dive. Only a fool never feels afraid underwater.

On most jobs, if the work is complex, divers will be trained in the operation of the specific tools they will be expected to use prior to the start of the job. However, if the tools are simple or familiar, there may be times where a diver does not see or use the tool until he is underwater. For example, one of the authors made a series of 380-foot saturation dives from a drill rig in the Gulf of Mexico to perform maintenance on a blow-out preventer stack (a device used to control an oil well during the exploratory drilling phase). On the first dive, he was required to cut away a series of broken guide wires used to lower the "stack" to the bottom. A hydraulic cable cutter was lowered to the diving bell to do the job. Although he had never seen or used the tool before, he immediately figured it out and used it successfully.

During the course of a dive, the diver should constantly communicate with the topside supervisor or rack operator. It is the diver's responsibility to let topside know exactly where he is at all times, and to keep the supervisor informed regarding the progress on the job.

Divers are paid a premium according to the depth of their dive. The pay scale varies from company to company, but the normal scale is that for dives to 50 feet or less the diver receives no additional pay. Beyond 50 feet, there is normally a bonus

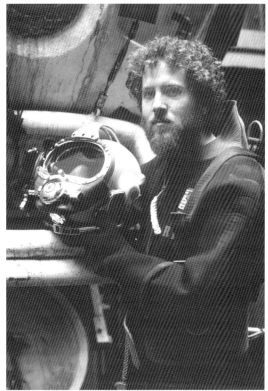

Fig. 13.8 Divers must be confident without being "cocky."

for each additional foot of depth. Divers who enter saturation may receive "pressure pay" where they are compensated for every hour they spend under pressure.

Diver–Tenders

The job classification of diver-tender is, as its name implies, an intermediate job category for employees who have more experience and skill than an entry level tender, but who have not yet been promoted to diver. In many cases, a person who has been advanced to diver-tender status is considered ready to promote to diver, but there are no slots in the company open for another diver.

Tenders

In the commercial diving field, the "tender," or apprentice, is the entry-level position at which most companies hire graduates of commercial diving schools.

Despite the fact that there are standards for commercial diving, every company uses equipment that is slightly different and will have their own procedures and policies. It takes time for a new tender to learn how the company does things, and to work smoothly as part of a team. Additionally, students at commercial diving schools don't get enough diving experience under real world conditions to enable them to be productive divers when they are first hired.

Tenders start out working on deck. Among the many responsibilities a tender may have while working on deck are:

• Fueling all deck machinery including compressors, hydraulic systems, welding machines, and other equipment.

• Dressing and tending the diver.

• Lowering tools and equipment to the diver on the bottom.

• Running the decompression chamber following surface-oriented dives.

• Performing maintenance on equipment.

• Launching and recovering the diving bell during saturation operations.

Properly dressing and tending the diver is the single most important responsibility the tender is assigned. He must ensure that the diver has donned his gear properly, that all of the connections between the hoses and cables are correctly made, and that the diver is kept comfortable while he stands by for his turn to dive.

While the diver is in the water, the tender must maintain a firm grip on the divers hose and keep a watchful eye for any activity that could pose a threat to the diver. The tender takes his direction from the diving supervisor or rack-operator, with whom he is in constant communication, either visually or by some type of audible communications system.

The tender must only provide hose to the diver when it is requested and must reel in the diver's excess hose promptly when instructed to do so. Too much slack hose in the water can be dangerous, especially if it becomes entangled in equipment on the bottom. This hazard increases in situations where there is a strong current.

Some hard-working tenders get their first opportunity to dive soon after they are hired, although most of their early dives will be in shallow water. Deeper dives that are paid a depth premium are

Risk Recognition for Divers and Diving Professionals

Commercial diving operations normally have a clear-cut chain of command, but few commercial companies take the time to rehearse what to do when an accident occurs. In the commercial environment, pressure is always present to get the job done as quickly as possible. Since most commercial companies are not located on waterfront property, the opportunity to practice for an emergency is not usually readily available.

On a long-term operation, however, there is usually sufficient down time for every dive team to practice emergency drills and analyze how to improve their response time. The value of this type of practice cannot be over-emphasized, particularly given the difficulty of recovering a diver into a diving bell or back aboard most larger vessels.

Another problem that faces most larger commercial firms is the fact that divers and tenders move from job to job in the same company, so that a team that has practiced their emergency skills together on one job will not usually be together on the next job. In addition, if the company uses "vessels of opportunity" the procedures for handling an incident may vary widely from one ship to the next.

normally reserved for divers or diver-tenders. Most companies have little expectation for a tender's early dives to be productive.

If a tender does well during his first few dives he will usually find himself working as part of the diving "rotation" for surface-supplied dives. If he continues to do well, demonstrating the right attitude and abilities, he will be promoted to diver-tender, sometimes within the first year of his employment.

Teamwork is an important part of any commercial diving operation. While divers are usually very tolerant of individual quirks or eccentricities, there is little tolerance for someone who doesn't carry their share of the load or places others at risk. A tender who is not compatible with others is usually off the job in short order.

Tenders normally serve an apprenticeship of anywhere from one to four years, depending on the size of the dive company and the amount of work for which the company has contracted. However, during the boom periods in the diving industry, particularly in the offshore environment, tenders may be promoted to diver status much more quickly. In some instances, tenders in these situations have been promoted before they have sufficient experience to work safely underwater.

Tenders are often in a position to directly observe any topside factors that may have contributed to the accident, although a new tender may not always understand what they have seen.

Dive Team Size

Generally speaking, the size of the dive crew will relate directly to the water depth of the job, i.e., the deeper the job, the more personnel will be required. However, shallow water jobs that are large or require round-the-clock diving may have larger crews than what the water depth would normally dictate.

The minimum size dive team that the

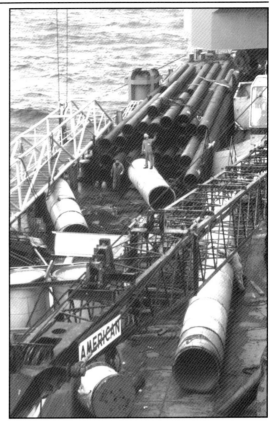

Fig. 13.9 In the offshore environment the work goes on 24 hours a day.

ADCI recommends for a shallow water diving job is a three-man team composed of a diver and two tenders. The rationale behind this size team is that a single tender would not be able to go to the aid of a diver who was incapacitated underwater.

OSHA requires three men on an air diving job, including a "designated person in charge" (diving supervisor), a diver, and a tender.

On a job that is within the range of air diving (down to 190 FSW, or 220 FSW for up to 30 minutes) the size of the crew will usually be anywhere from four to six (or more) people. The complexity of the job and the amount of decompression required for each diver will determine the manpower needs.

A surface-supplied mixed-gas diving job will usually require a crew of at least twelve men, if there is any complexity

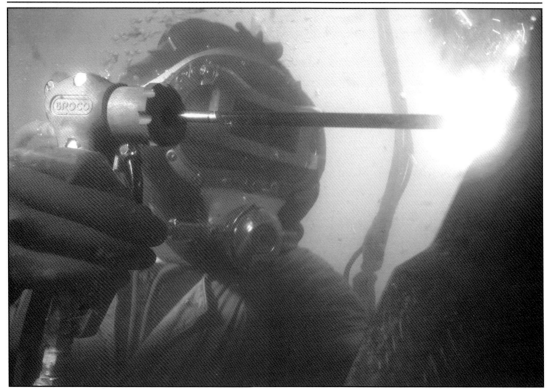

Fig. 13.10 Each different underwater task presents unique hazards and a Job Hazard Analysis should be performed before any work. Cutting with an arc-oxygen underwater torch can lead to an explosion with life threatening potential if proper procedures are not followed.

to the job at all. On a saturation diving job in deep water, the normal crew size will usually be 24 people. This allows for a team of six divers in saturation, for round-the-clock diving, and enough crew on deck to conduct surface oriented diving if needed.

The investigator should obtain the name of every person on the job and secure a statement from each person who has direct knowledge of the incident.

The Job–Site Environment

On a large diving job, with a round-the-clock crew, the normal workday is a 12-hour shift for all personnel. In most cases there is a night crew that works from midnight till noon and a day crew that works from noon until midnight. Obviously, some people adapt better to this situation than others, but for some the interruption of a normal sleep pattern can be disruptive. When changes in personnel dictate that a crewmember change

from the day shift to the night shift, this type of change can be unsettling, too.

On smaller jobs where a diving crew is called to do emergency repairs on an offshore structure or inland operation, the work may proceed round-the-clock with one crew, until the project is completed or additional personnel arrive. Fatigue and disorientation can affect the entire crews' performance.

Even in situations where the crew works a normal shift, some offshore installations have inadequate sleeping quarters so that other workers may be disturbing the sleep of the diving crew. In some cases, divers are given the least preferred accommodations, such as a cabin located near running machinery or other sources of noise.

Success as a commercial diver, particularly in the oilfield, usually requires a person to spend long periods of time offshore. A typical personnel rotation on an offshore job requires thirty days at sea, followed by ten days of leave, in the offshore oilfield environment. "Boom" periods have occurred during the development of new oilfields, like the North Sea, or following powerful hurricanes where offshore installations have been heavily damaged or destroyed. During these times, there can be tremendous pressure on divers to work for extended periods offshore, with little or no leave.

Emotional stress is quite often a factor in the lives of divers who spend long periods of time offshore, particularly for those who have families or are engaged in committed relationships. The old joke about divers being located right next to "divorce" in the telephone directory is not too far from the truth.

Most divers do not work offshore for more than five or six years because of the lifestyle. The psychological stress of the environment, as well as the lifestyle, can lead to less than optimal performance by some members of the dive crew.

As you investigate a commercial diving accident, you should gently probe to see if any of these issues played a role in affecting the performance of the crewmembers involved.

Job Hazard Analysis (JHA)

In an attempt to help reduce the risks of each diving job, the ADCI has included the performance of a Job Hazard Analysis (JHA) by the diving supervisor prior to the start of any new underwater work project. The JHA is designed to make the supervisor and the rest of the crew cognizant of any dangers that may occur during the operation and to implement whatever safety measures are necessary before a problem can occur.

During the JHA the supervisor and crew break the job down into its individual tasks and determine the dangers involved in each step. The crew then determines what actions are needed to minimize or eliminate these risks. The JHA should be recorded and filed with the other job paperwork.

Whenever investigating a commercial accident, ask the diving supervisor if he performed a JHA and if he has a written copy of what was covered in the analysis. You should examine this document to determine if the supervisor anticipated the factors that caused the accident and what steps were taken in an attempt to avoid the situation.

Company Safety Manual

Each diving company is required by OSHA and the USCG to have a diving safety manual to cover its operations. A copy of this manual should be available on each job site. The manual covers the policies and procedures used by the company to help maintain a safe working environment.

Review a copy of the company's safety manual to see which aspects of it pertain to the accident you are investigating .

Record Keeping

According to U.S. Coast Guard and OSHA standards, commercial diving companies must also regularly test and inspect their equipment. These inspections include hoses, chambers, gauges, air supplies, etc. The results of these tests must be recorded and maintained in the company's files. You should review these records to confirm the maintenance and performance of any equipment that was involved in an accident.

In addition to the equipment records, the company is also required to keep a copy of the log for each dive, as well as the diving physical exams for each individual person who works in the field. Examine the dive logs of any diver who is injured or killed on the job, as well as his physical exam records. You only need to see the dive logs from the dives made on the job where the incident occurred.

Since physical exam records are considered personal information, an attorney may need to subpoena these documents.

Use of Rental Equipment by Commercial Companies

In many cases, a diving company may not have all of the equipment it needs to do a large or specialized job. It's common for diving contractors to rent equipment. This is particularly true for small contractors, but large companies will sometimes need to rent gear to complete a job, too.

The most commonly rented equipment will normally be specialized tools, such as a waterblaster or cutting saw, that the company does not need on a daily basis. Occasionally diving companies will also rent decompression chambers, compressors, or other diving equipment.

One of the things to check for when you investigate a commercial diving accident will be to determine if any of the equipment used on the job was rented or leased and if it played a role in the accident. It may be more difficult to obtain maintenance records from an outside firm, and in most cases you will need a subpoena to obtain this type of information.

Types of Commercial Diving Accidents

There are many different types of commercial diving accidents. However, certain types of accidents seem to occur regularly, due to the inherent dangers of the occupation.

Most divers acknowledge and accept the risks involved in their profession, but normally try to minimize the risks. For some, the danger is part of what makes the job interesting and exciting.

Some of the commercial diving accidents that occur are simply construction accidents that could happen on any job site, but when they happen to a diver, the incident becomes a diving accident. Other types of accidents are peculiar to commercial diving and do not happen in other environments.

Construction Accidents

When a heavy object is dropped at a construction site, people don't always have time to get out of the way. On many commercial diving jobs, the underwater visibility is so poor that it would be impossible for the diver to see any object falling through the water. In addition, a diver can't swim quickly and even if he could, the object might land on his hose. If a heavy object lands on the divers hose it can pinch off the diver's air supply or completely sever the hose.

Heavy objects have on occasion crushed divers underwater. In another instance, a diver surfaced between a barge and a boat and was actually saved by his helmet, which resisted the impact between the two vessels when they came together.

Polluted Water

Many commercial diving jobs take place in polluted water. However, in numerous situations, the divers do not realize that this is the case, or just ignore the issue. Although it's rare for a diver to die shortly after exposure to polluted water, many divers have experienced long term illnesses. A recent study by an Israeli doctor, Dr. Elihu Richter documents cases of cancer in Israeli Navy divers after repeated exposures to polluted water environments (*Richter, 2002*).

The two main types of pollutants that divers typically encounter are biological hazards and chemical hazards. In many bodies of water, both types of hazards are present.

To dive properly in polluted water, divers must wear vulcanized rubber dry suits, with a helmet and gloves that attach directly to the suit. The helmet must be equipped with a special double exhaust valve to prevent contaminants from entering the helmet through the diver's breathing system.

Following a dive in polluted water, the diver must be properly decontaminated before removing his dry suit. This type of operation must be planned in advance and requires extensive support.

Divers can be protected from virtually any type of biological hazard, but there are some types of pollutants for which there is no adequate protection. There is no one type of diving suit or helmet that is compatible with all chemicals. In some polluted water environments, it is better to use an ROV (Remotely Operated Vehicle) than to use a diver.

Explosions

Commercial divers frequently use explosives underwater to cut through rock to lay pipelines or cables, or to salvage structures. Explosives are a quick way to cut through large amounts of material.

If a diver is in close proximity to an explosion underwater, the results may be fatal. The shock wave from an explosion underwater can be just as devastating as a shock wave topside.

One common type of explosive accident that can occur takes place when a diver is engaged in underwater cutting or "burning" using an arc-oxygen cutting torch. The torch is supplied with electrical power and oxygen from topside via a cable and hose.

The arc-oxygen torch uses a hollow electrode that is consumed as the diver makes the cut. A ground cable is connected to the work to complete the circuit. When the power is switched on to the torch, tremendous heat is produced at the tip of the electrode where it touches the metal. When the diver pulls the trigger on the torch, oxygen flows through the electrode to the tip of the torch and the base metal on the structure to be cut literally "burns." An experienced diver using an oxy-arc torch can make extremely precise cuts in steel structures in a relatively short time.

During the "burning" process, the arc-oxygen (or "oxy-arc") torch also liberates hydrogen from the water. When the diver is cutting in open water, this is not a problem. However, if a diver is cutting inside a closed compartment, such as inside a ship or a pipe, hydrogen can accumulate at the top of the compartment, as well as any oxygen that is not consumed as part of the burning process. If the diver has not taken the precaution to cut a vent hole in the compartment, a spark from the torch can ignite the mixture and cause an explosion. More than one diver has been killed this way.

Waterblaster Accidents

High-pressure water blasters are useful tools used to clean hard growth or paint off of marine structures. This type of equipment is designed to deliver a high-speed jet of water at pressures of up to 10,000 pounds per square inch. The system consists of a topside pump with a long hose that connects the pump to the waterblaster "gun" or nozzle used by the diver underwater. The stream of water delivered by this type of equipment can easily cut through diving suits and human flesh.

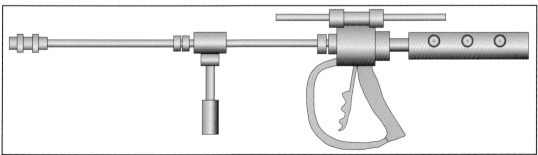

Fig. 13.11 Waterblasters can produce painful wounds that are readily subject to infection.

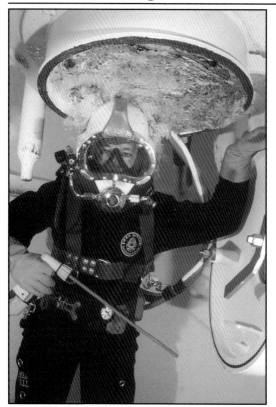

Fig. 13.12 If a diving bell is lost while the divers are on the bottom, recovery can be a difficult operation.

There have been several accidents that have occurred when divers have been using high-pressure water blasters and accidentally ran the blaster over their foot. This is an extremely dangerous type of accident because the blaster almost always injects bacteria into the tissue of the foot, which can lead to a serious infection if not treated promptly.

Divers using high-pressure water blasters underwater should be equipped with either steel-toed boots or meta-tarsal guards like those used for topside protection. Like any tool, waterblasters should only be used for their intended purpose, and not for tasks such as washing away loose mud.

Pressure Differential

Divers can be trapped or injured underwater when a pressure differential occurs in close proximity, but external to the divers body. For example, if a diver is working on a dam, and a valve is opened underwater that vents to surface pressure, the diver can be sucked against the valve and held against it. If the valve opening is large enough and the pressure is great enough, the differential can sever an arm or a leg.

Under situations where there are valves that could produce any suction, such as a seawater intake on an oil platform or ship, the valve should be "red-tagged," and preferably physically "locked out" of use, if there are divers working underwater. There must be a warning sign placed over the valve that there are divers working in the water. Ideally, there should also be a member of the dive crew stationed at the valve to ensure that no one from the ship's crew ignores the warning on the valve and opens it anyway.

If this type of accident occurs, you should check what steps were taken to lock the valve out of use. Be sure to photograph the location of the valve and identify it in the photograph.

Many commercial diving accidents have been caused by pressure differentials. In one case, the diver's leg was sucked into an eight inch diameter pipe and the pipe had to be cut to free the diver. The diver was brought to the surface with a section of pipe still attached to his leg.

Lost Bell

For a diver making a bell-bounce or saturation dive, one of the most dangerous accidents that can occur happens when the lift wire and umbilical for the bell are severed from the ship so that bell and the divers are trapped on the bottom. When this occurs, the greatest danger to the divers is that they will die from hypothermia, since there is no external supply of hot water to the diving bell. Some bells carry devices similar to sleeping bags that the divers can enter to help conserve body heat. However, without any warming for the breathing gas in the bell environment, heat loss will still be high.

Diving bells should be equipped with electronic locating devices known as "pingers" that can be used to locate a lost bell on the bottom. Devices like these can significantly increase the likelihood of a successful rescue.

There are two major problems that limit the likelihood of a successful rescue of a lost bell. In situations where the bell is lost at water depths in excess of 400 feet, it is extremely hazardous to make a dive to effect the recovery of the bell without another bell system to perform the job. A solitary surface-supplied diver is at great risk at these depths if anything goes wrong during the dive.

The other major problem in rescuing a lost bell is that even if the bell is recovered, unless there is another diving system in the vicinity with exactly the same type of mating system for the bell, the decompression of divers must be completed in the bell itself. While it's relatively easy to re-establish connections for life support to the bell, in most cases, there's no way to get food into the divers or lock human wastes out of the bell. Additionally, due to the relatively small size of most diving bells, the divers will usually be forced to maintain cramped postures inside the bell, which may compromise their decompression.

When the drop weights are ditched by the divers in the bell, the bell should, theoretically rise to the surface. The insulating foam used on the exterior of most bells, known as "syntactic foam," should provide sufficient buoyancy to lift the bell to the surface. However, if the lift wire for the bell broke near the surface, the bell could be entangled on the bottom by its own lift wire. In this case, the divers would need to lock out of the bell, without hot water, to cut away the wire.

Fortunately, the number of circumstances when diving bells have been lost

are relatively rare, but the potential for this type of accident is always present. A near-miss of this type occurred in the North Sea, when the bell was dragged through a platform as its support vessel accidentally shifted its position. The bell tipped on its side, flooding the interior, and the lift wire came close to snapping. Only the teamwork of the diving crew topside saved the bell divers from an extremely serious accident.

Contaminated Breathing Air

The possibility of a diver receiving carbon monoxide laden air has already been discussed in Chapter 4, but any toxic chemical fumes that are pumped to the diver can cause an accident. In addition, even if the diver's air compressor has been properly set up and installed on the job, if another internal combustion system is operating upwind from the diver's compressor, the chance of delivering carbon monoxide to the diver exists. This type of incident might occur on a barge or oil platform if other workers who are

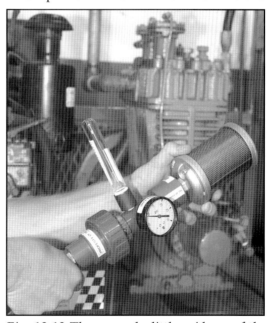

Fig. 13.13 There may be little evidence of the presence of contaminated air in a low pressure compressor system unless the investigation takes place within a short time of this type of accident.

not part of the dive crew set up a diesel driven welding machine or other machinery in close proximity to the diver's air compressor.

It can be difficult to establish the cause of death in this type of situation unless you are on the scene within a short time of the incident. If the compressor or other machinery is moved, there may be little or no evidence that will point to the cause of the contamination of the breathing air. In addition, due to the limited amount of air in most compressor volume tanks, unless the volume tank is sealed immediately following the incident, there may be little or no trace of contamination in the system.

Saturation System Failures

Although it's unusual, occasionally some component of a saturation system will fail, and cause a life-threatening situation. The biggest danger to the diver in this type of situation is rapid depressurization of the system, which could expose the diver to explosive decompression.

In most cases, rapid decompression of a saturation diver will cause death.

In some cases, saturation system failures have occurred when crewmembers have installed the wrong component as part of the diving system. For example, if a valve with an insufficient pressure rating was installed as part of the system, this could lead to a breakdown of the equipment.

In one particularly horrific accident, the mating flange that connected a diving bell to the trunk on an entrance lock on a saturation system failed and the entire system experienced rapid decompression. Several divers died in this tragic accident.

Commercial Diving Accidents Involving Boats

In commercial diving accidents, it's rare for the diver to be injured by the boat from which he was operating, but it does occur. It is much more common for a diver to be injured by a boat moving through the area where the diver was working.

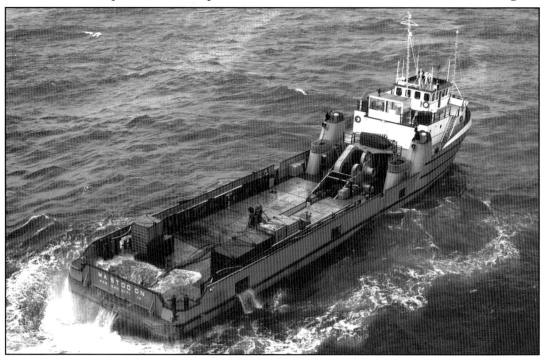

Fig. 13.14 Since many types of vessels play an intricate role in the work of commercial divers, accidents are almost inevitable in this environment.

What Happens When a Boat Snags a Diver's Hose

As we've already mentioned in the section on commercial seafood divers, it's possible for a commercial diver's hose to be snagged by a boat moving through the dive site. Although this is a common accident with floating hose, most inshore and oilfield divers use sinking hose, so this type of accident is less common among these types of divers.

In circumstances involving larger vessels, the divers hose may be severed or be wound up in the prop. If the diver's hose is severed, the diver will be forced to make an emergency ascent to the surface, which could lead to decompression sickness. If the diver's hose is wound up in the prop, the diver could be dragged into or through underwater structures, which could result in physical injury or unconsciousness, which may lead to drowning. If the diver is dragged into the ship's propeller, he could be severely cut or experience severed limbs.

Commercial divers often engage in a type of diving procedure known as "liveboating," where the diver walks along a pipeline or other structure underwater, and the vessel from which he is being tended follows behind him. With an inexperienced tender or boat skipper, or under rough seas, the diver's own support vessel could run over his hose, precipitating an accident.

Accidents Involving Dynamically Positioned Vessels

Dynamically positioned vessels are ships that do not anchor, but have multiple thrusters, both fore and aft ship, that maintain the vessel in one location. The thrusters are controlled by a computer system that maintains the vessel in a (theoretically) precise location by sensing the vessels location relative to a set of transponders in the water or to GPS satellites. Dynamically positioned vessels are sometimes referred to as "DP" vessels, as a shorthand name.

Most diving from a DP vessel is relatively incident free. However, if the DP system fails for any reason, the ship may move rapidly away from its desired location. If this happens while a diver is underwater, the diver could be seriously injured or killed, especially if the diver was working inside a wreck or other underwater structure when the vessel starts to move.

As an investigator, you should determine how the DP system operated and whether it was functioning properly. In most cases, a separate expert in this area will probably make that determination. However, you should examine the communication between the ship's crew and the diving supervisor.

Jones Act Seaman Status

The Jones Act is a U.S. maritime law originally written in 1920. The intent of the law was to provide a way for a ship's crew member to receive financial compensation in the event an individual was injured while at sea. When a person is injured at sea and the law determines that the individual was a Jones Act Seaman, the financial award that can be provided to an individual exceeds what that person might receive otherwise. For this reason, a plaintiff's attorney will usually be anxious to prove that his client was a Jones Act Seaman, while the defense will vigorously assert that the circumstances do not support such a claim.

To determine whether a person is a Jones Act Seaman or not the law applies several "tests" to the facts of a case. To qualify as a Jones Act seaman the conditions that must be met are as follows:

• The person who is injured must be working on the vessel to further the work that is being performed by the vessel and its crew **and** the vessel must be "in navigation" (mobile). A diver who works only on fixed (anchored into the bottom) offshore platforms, or on stationary barges, would not qualify as a Jones Act Seaman.

• The diver must have a relationship or "attachment" with the vessel in navigation, i.e., he cannot be a "freelance" diver who jumps from company to company. He must make a substantial portion of his living working offshore for the same company (i.e., greater than 30% of his time must be spent in the service of a vessel in navigation.)

Another issue that the court will examine is whether the vessel is part of a fleet of vessels owned by the company or whether this is an individual vessel. If the diver worked aboard different vessels that were part of the fleet for the same company, the court will be more disposed to consider the diver a Jones Act seaman. The definition of what constitutes a vessel may be quite broad, and in one case

an attempt was made to characterize a surfboard as a "vessel."

If the diver is not considered a Jones Act Seaman by the court, then he will usually fall under the Longshore and Harbor Worker's Compensation Act. Under this section of the law, the compensation to the diver or his heirs might be less.

Your job as an investigator assisting an attorney on a case that may be a potential Jones Act situation will be to provide the facts of the case and not an interpretation of the law. You will need to check on the diver's work history with the diving company and the attorneys will evaluate this information in light of the law.

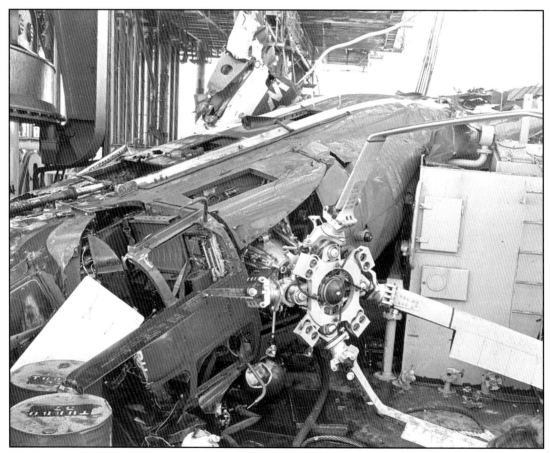

Fig. 13.15 When this helicopter crashed onto a North Sea barge, it barely missed the saturation diving system on deck. See the case history on the next page. (Photo © Gary Beyerstein.)

Case History – Commercial Oilfield Diving

Back in the mid-70s, at the height of the North Sea oil boom, there were hundreds of divers working offshore in the waters between the UK, Norway and Holland. The exploration of potential new oil fields and the construction of new platforms was occurring at a breakneck pace.

One of the barges that operated in the British sector for an extended period of time was the *Thor*. This massive construction vessel had a huge permanently mounted crane, scores of riggers and construction workers, and a full-time complement of divers. The barge stayed offshore for months at a time, in some of the worst weather imaginable. The *Thor* was instrumental in the construction and development of the Forties Field, one of the major developments owned by British Petroleum (BP).

Workers, mail, and small items were shuttled out to the *Thor* and the surrounding platforms by helicopter on a daily basis. With the Forties Field lying several hundred miles offshore, helicopter transportation was the fastest, most efficient way to move critical manpower.

The diving system aboard the *Thor* was a full saturation system that could house six divers at a time. The system was in constant use as construction went on around the clock, whenever weather permitted. The average diving depth in the Forties Field was 400 FSW and the divers were instrumental in the development of the area's oil resources.

One day, the *Thor* was moored right next to one of the platforms as the crew worked on one of the many tasks involved in bringing the oilfield on-line. As the crew worked on the structure below the accommodations on the platform, another crew worked on the decks of the platform itself.

A helicopter landed on the platform, the relief crew disembarked and the previous crew boarded the aircraft. As the chopper took off, it suddenly lost power, and began to fall towards the barge. On the deck of the *Thor*, workers scattered in all directions.

To the crew caring for the divers in the saturation system, it appeared that the aircraft was going to hit the sat system, or the oxygen cylinders right next to it. In either case, it would have been a major catastrophe for the divers. If it had hit the chambers, it would almost have certainly compromised their integrity, exposing the divers to explosive decompression. If it had hit the oxygen cylinders, the resulting fire and explosions could have been equally damaging to the saturation diving system.

Fortunately for the divers, the helicopter missed both the chambers and the oxygen supply, but still crashed on the deck of the barge. Although there was no explosion, most of the barge crew were hesitant to move close to the downed aircraft and stayed back, waiting for someone to take action to get the injured men out of the fuselage. Interestingly, only the divers who were working on the deck of the barge came forward to drag the injured men out of the helicopter.

This could have been a much more serious incident had the saturation system been damaged. What is interesting to note is that like many of the accidents that involve divers in the oilfield, the root cause has nothing to do with diving itself, but involves some other aspect of the offshore construction environment.

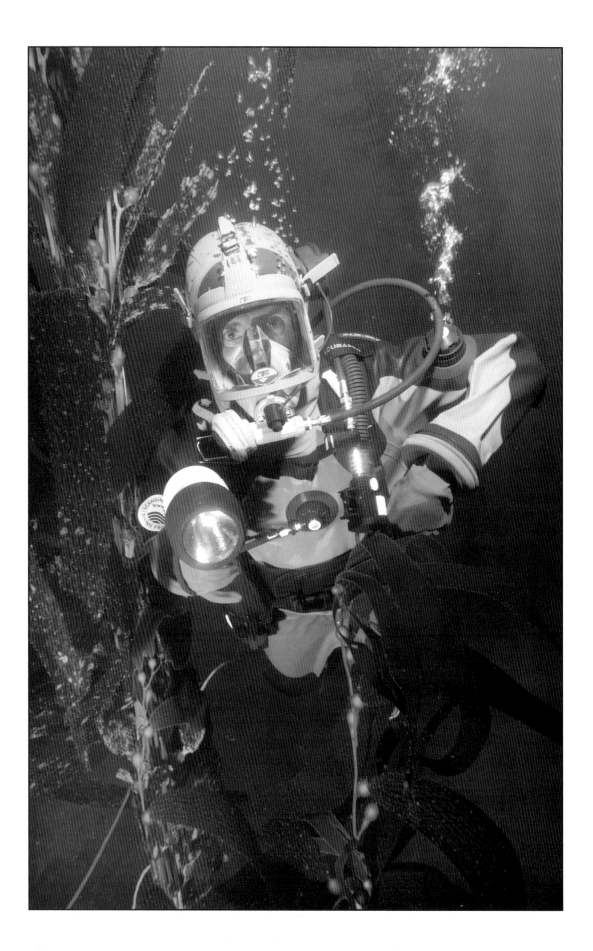

Chapter 14
Preparing Your Report and Testimony

At the end of the day, your client or employer will almost invariably expect you to prepare some type of written report detailing the accident. It is your job to write the report so that people who are not familiar with diving will understand what took place. It's crucial that you explain any unfamiliar terms and do not allow yourself to use jargon.

If you're writing a report for a law enforcement agency, you'll undoubtedly have a standard report format that must be followed. However, if you are writing a report for an attorney or insurance company, there will likely be no standard format and you will need to develop your own. In this chapter, we'll take a look at some of the different types of information that should be included to produce a detailed report.

Remember that your job is to report the facts of the case and not to speculate (unless you have specifically been instructed to do so) on what took place. Do not include your opinions in the report. Do not include commentary on matters which you are not qualified to comment on.

Interpreting Documents

Your report will usually include documents from any number of agencies. It's important to read these reports carefully and with a healthy degree of skepticism. Not everything in these documents will be true, and existing data may be open to multiple interpretations. To piece together an accurate picture of what occurred, you must evaluate and correlate the information from each document to write a coherent report.

Most of the law enforcement and rescue agency reports will be quite straightforward. However, there may be inaccurate observations or interpretations of what took place, based on the knowledge and background of the person writing the report. Law enforcement and rescue agencies may use abbreviations or shorthand that may be hard to understand if you are not familiar with it.

Understanding the Autopsy

The most difficult document to understand will usually be the autopsy. You should have access to a medical dictionary that defines any terms you might not know. Another handy document is a drug identification book, such as the Physician's Desk Reference (PDR) so that you understand the use and side effects of any prescription drugs the victim might have been taking. The autopsy will usually include the following:

• A description of the physical aspects of the body including height, weight, unusual body features, as well as measurements and descriptions of the internal organs.

• An interpretation by the coroner of the results of the forensic examination.

• A toxicology report (or "tox" for

Orange County Sheriff-Coroner
Forensic Science Services / Toxicology Laboratory
Report of Toxicological Examination

FR NUMBER: ███████   CORONER CASE NUMBER: ███████

NAME OF DECEASED: ███████

INVESTIGATOR: ███████   AGE: 50   SEX: Male

SPECIMENS SUBMITTED: ☑ Postmortem Blood   ☐ Brain   ☐ Stomach Contents   ☐ Urine
                      ☐ Antemortem Samples   ☐ Liver   ☐ Vitreous Humor   ☐ Peripheral Blood

Other Specimens: None

BLOOD RECEIVED BY: Herndon   FROM: Tkocs
TISSUE RECEIVED BY: FROM:

Page 1 of 1

Findings

Drug	Matrix	Method	Result	Anal	Anal
Ephedrine/Pseudoephedrine	Postmortem Blood	GC/MS	Detected	WBE	SCW
Norpseudoephedrine	Postmortem Blood	GC/MS	Detected	WBE	SCW

Analyses

Drug	Matrix	Method	Result	Anal	Anal
Ethanol/Volatiles	Postmortem Blood	Headspace/GC	None Detected	ARG	MXS
Cocaine Metabolite	Postmortem Blood	Immunoassay	Negative	LXW	
Phenethylamines	Postmortem Blood	Immunoassay	See Findings	LXW	
Opiates	Postmortem Blood	Immunoassay	Negative	LXW	
Barbiturates	Postmortem Blood	Immunoassay	Negative	LXW	
Amphetamine/Methamphetamine	Postmortem Blood	GC/MS	None Detected	WBE	SCW
Amphetamine Related Stimulants	Postmortem Blood	GC/MS	See Findings	WBE	SCW

Fig. 14.1 The toxicology report may be crucial to understanding the accident.

short) which normally will not include any interpretation of the findings.

• An official cause of death.

It's not uncommon for a coroner to make unwarranted assumptions in dive accident cases. You should watch carefully for this type of error as you read through a coroner's report. Coroners often receive information about the circumstances of the accident that is incorrect. Coroners who are not knowledgeable about diving sometimes fail to document air in the chest cavity or vascular system, even in accidents that are obvious cases of arterial gas embolism.

If you are an insurance investigator and are in contact with the coroner, do not attend the autopsy even if you are invited to do so. This opens you up to possible charges of bias and tampering with a witness.

If there is something about the autopsy that is not clear, see if you can find information on the topic in a medical text or on the Internet. If the findings are still unclear, you may call the coroner to see if he will explain his report. Keep in mind, however, that as an investigator, your job is not to interpret medical opinions but to collect information and present facts.

Sometimes you'll find information in an autopsy that you know is wrong. If you are a law enforcement officer, you may want to tactfully contact the coroner to discuss these issues with the examiner. Otherwise, if you are an outsider to the local law enforcement community, limit your findings of any errors to your report.

Unfortunately, errors in the autopsy report are extremely common. Furthermore, coroners often have little knowledge of diving, diving practices, diving equipment, and diving physiology. It is entirely possible for an experienced investigator to know more about the physiology of a diving fatality than a medical examiner.

There are a variety of errors in medical examiner's reports that show up with some frequency. The most common error is for a death to be ascribed to drowning when the circumstances of the death would suggest another cause. For example, drowning is a perfectly understandable explanation for a death when a diver gets trapped in a cave and runs out of air. On the other hand, drowning is a nonsensical diagnosis for a diver swimming back to the dive boat or back to shore who suddenly dies. It is important to realize that at autopsy, there are no specific findings to prove the diagnosis of drowning. However, there are findings that can disprove the diagnosis of drowning, i.e., normal weight of the lungs. As a result, the diagnosis of drowning should be made on the basis of compatible autopsy findings and a sequence of events consistent with a drowning. If the medical examiner does otherwise it may be appropriate to factually point this out in the investigative report.

To further complicate matters, there are a variety of conditions that can occur to a diver which can cause him to drown. Thus, an oxygen induced convulsion from breathing a gas mixture too rich in oxygen may cause a diver to drown when the operational cause of death was the gas mix. Similarly, an AGE (arterial

---

COUNTY OF LOS ANGELES

THOMAS T. NOGUCHI, M.D.
CHIEF MEDICAL EXAMINER-CORONER

12 AUTOPSY REPORT

No.   -13136

I performed an autopsy on the body of ➡

at ___ the DEPARTMENT OF CHIEF MEDICAL EXAMINER—CORONER

Los Angeles, California   on OCTOBER 23, 1983 @ 1100 HOURS
                               (Date)   (Time)

From the anatomic findings and pertinent history I ascribe the death to:

(A)   DROWNING

DUE TO OR AS A CONSEQUENCE OF
(B)
DUE TO OR AS A CONSEQUENCE OF
(C)
OTHER SIGNIFICANT CONDITIONS—

Anatomical Summary:

1.   Presence of air bubbles in the heart, in the aorta, and in the inferior vena cava.

2.   Pulmonary edema and congestion, marked (right 700 grams, left 690 grams).

3.   Cerebral edema (1,600 grams) dusky cortex, the white matter shows presence of petechiae, marked congestion of the subarachnoid, meningeal and dural vessels.

4.   No traumatic injuries.

5.   No other focal lesions in any of the organs.

Fig. 14.2 Autopsy reports are not always correct in their conclusions. As a dive accident investigator, you must read them carefully.

gas embolism) can result in a diver losing consciousness and then drowning. At autopsy there may be nothing to specifically indicate that a seizure or an AGE was the underlying factor in the death of the diver. It is the investigator's job to gather enough data to be able to interpret the death in a cogent manner. It is for this reason that stool in a dry suit or a tank with the valve only opened a quarter of a turn becomes critical information.

Death due to a cardiac event in the water also may not have any specific findings at the autopsy. Such a death can easily be misinterpreted as a drowning.

Again, it may be the sequence of events and the pattern of circumstances that are most important in establishing the cause of death. This is the province of the investigator and all too often, medical examiners are unaware of, or ignore, these events and circumstances.

Autopsies may be anywhere from half a dozen pages to almost 50 pages, depending on the case. Read the autopsy carefully and look for any unusual issues that you may need to investigate further or that should be highlighted in your final report.

Risk Recognition for Divers and Diving Professionals

In the event your are present during a diving accident, it's imperative that you respond to the incident in a responsible and professional manner, not just during the incident itself, but also in the days, weeks, and months following it. Your actions subsequent to the incident may be as important as what you do at the time of the accident.

Prior to leaving the accident site, be sure you have the names, phone numbers, and addresses of everyone who was present at the time of the event. If the equipment has not been impounded by the police, lock up any items that were worn by the diver.

One of the first issues that you will invariably need to address will be the inquiries from reporters who want to know what happened. Do not make any suppositions or even suggest a version of the incident. Despite the fact that you were there, do not be tempted to talk at length about the incident. There will almost always be many things that you don't know about the accident, such as whether the victim was under the influence of drugs, the condition of the diving equipment at the moment of the accident, and other specifics.

Give a polite but short response, such as, "We don't know all the facts about the incident at this time." Avoid answering any detailed questions beyond the basics, such as the name of the boat, the approximate time of day, or the location.

Once you have called your insurance company, sit down and write down everything that you know about the incident (if you have not already done so). Store this information (as well as any photos or video that may have been shot that day) in a secure location, such as a safe deposit box.

Be prepared to fully cooperate with the accident investigator from your insurance company. Do not withhold any information from him.

Be kind and considerate to the family of the victim. Treat them the way you would like to be treated if the victim was someone related to you. Again, even if you think you know what happened, do not ascribe blame. There is no way you can know all the facts.

Do not be tempted to enter into conversations about what took place with other divers, on the Internet, or in any other venue.

Date	Time	Event	Source
Oct. 2000		Smith completes Open Water I certification.	Course records
June 2001		Smith participates in trip to Catalina Island.	Store receipt
Aug. 2003		Pre-trip meeting for Sept. 2 Santa Cruz Island	Dive master
Sept. 2, 2003		Smith arrives at dive boat's dock.	Dive master
Sept. 3, 2003	0600	Dive boat departs for Santa Cruz Island	Dive master
	0900	Dive boat arrives at dive site	Jackson
	1015	Smith and Jones enter water together	estimated
	1030	Smith passes out on bottom	estimated
	1035	Jones surfaces unconscious	USCG log
	1038	Jackson calls U.S. Coast Guard on VHF	USCG log
	1045	U.S.C.G. helicopter launched	USCG log
	1050	Sheriffs dive team initiates response	USCG log
	1055	Dive boat reports Smith missing	USCG log
	1115	U.S.C.G on site	USCG log
	1230	Sheriff's divers make first search for Smith	USCG log
	1250	Jones recompressed at Catalina chamber	estimated
	2000	Jones exits chamber	estimated
Additional aerial and underwater searches are made for Smith after September 3.			
Sept. 5, 2003		Smith's body is recovered.	

Fig. 14.3 Creating a chronology is almost always helpful to understanding what took place.

Creating a List of Persons Involved

One of the most essential elements to be included in your report is a list of all persons who were directly involved with the incident. The list should include their name, their role in the incident, their address, and their home and business telephone numbers. This list will make it easy for anyone who must read your report to instantly understand who did what and to follow up with anyone involved.

Creating a Chronology

One of the most useful documents you can create in analyzing any diving accident is a chronology of exactly what took place, including where and when. For most accidents, the chronology will be a one or two page record that includes the date and time of each individual action that was taken, including the source of the information.

The chronology for a diving accident may start the night before the incident or even weeks before the mishap took place. For example, in a training accident, you may want to show the lapse in time between the last confined water training and the open water dive when the accident took place to better put the event in perspective. In a situation where the individual who experienced the accident was drinking or using recreational or prescription drugs the night before the event, you should include the time and location where these items were consumed.

When you create a chronology there will invariably be actions that took place at undetermined times and you will have to make your best estimate of when these events took place. This is where your experience as a diver will be vital in arriving at reasonable estimates for different actions taken by the divers involved in the accident.

There will invariably be discrepancies between the times recorded by emergency services personnel working for different agencies. There may even be differences in times logged by personnel from the same agency who are in the field, compared to the times noted by dispatchers who are computer based. As long as the times are in reasonable proximity to each other, there is usually no great cause for you to be alarmed or to warrant further investigation. However, if the times reported by one agency are significantly different from those given by another agency or individual you should try to determine why this is the case.

Time estimates from individuals who were directly involved with the incident are notoriously inaccurate. As you create your chronology, be sure to note anything that is an estimate by an individual who was involved in the case.

Be sure to take advantage of any dive logs provided by dive computers owned by people who were involved in the episode. These devices will provide highly accurate profiles of the time intervals the divers spent at specific depths during each phase of the dive(s).

Writing a Summary

Probably the most difficult part of creating your report will be writing a summary of the event based on the interviews you have conducted and the documents you have obtained. A typical narrative report might run anywhere from two to four single spaced, typewritten pages. The summary is used to piece together the facts from each different source to arrive at one coherent version of what transpired. This is the crux of your report, and everything else will be supplementary.

In most cases, you should place your summary towards the front of your report, (after the chronology), to allow anyone who reviews your document to quickly get a grasp of the facts of the case.

Writing the Gear Inspection

The basis for your report on the equipment inspection will be the gear inspection checklist that you used while conducting your investigation. In this section you include all of the observations you made while inspecting the equipment.

Compare the results of your examination of the equipment with the performance specifications for the equipment provided by the manufacturer. This is essential information for anyone who must review your findings.

The importance of not expressing your opinions in this section cannot be over-emphasized. For example, if you have strong feelings about the adequacy or performance of a piece of dive gear, you must put your personal beliefs aside and stick to the facts of the case. Your personal judgment about the poor design of a buoyancy compensator is not relevant to your report. What is relevant is the amount of lift that the BC provides relative to the amount of weight the diver was carrying on his belt and the buoyancy of his scuba cylinder and other accessories. Anything in your report should be factual and objective. There is no place in this type of document for your subjective beliefs or biases.

Include Photos and Drawings

Photos, drawings, and maps will help to improve the clarity of your report, provide additional information, and generally make the document more interesting to the reader. It's especially important to include photos that show any unusual features of a dive site or damage to a piece of equipment.

You should use some simple image editing software to highlight any important elements in your photos and label any important parts of the image. Circle

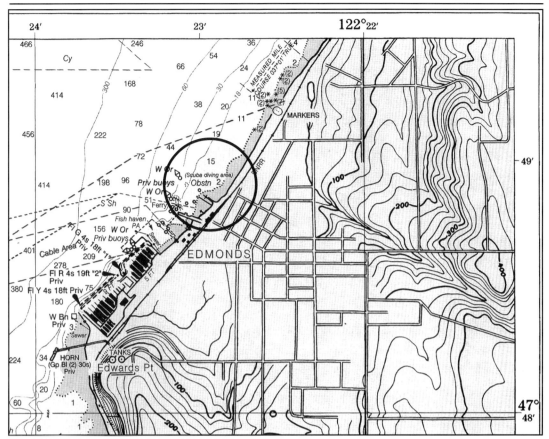

Fig. 14.4 If you can include both a chart of the site and a photograph, this will help to make it easier for the people who read your report to visualize what took place.

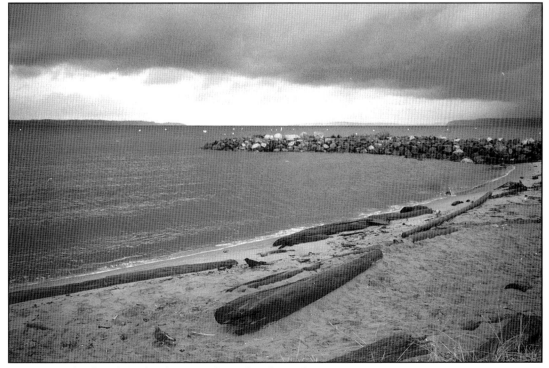

Fig. 14.5 This beach is the dive site from the chart above.

any key items in the photos or draw arrows that point to the objects to which you wish to draw the reader's attention.

Nautical charts are the best way to illustrate the location of the accident, and these should be included in every report. Street maps can also be used to identify the location of hospitals, emergency service providers, or other points of interest. These documents can be scanned into your computer and placed directly into your final document.

The Appendix

The appendix is the place to put copies of any documents that you have collected that will be helpful in evaluating the case, but may not be referenced in the body of the report itself. Documents that might be included in the appendix include the following:

- Training records
- Equipment maintenance records
- The autopsy
- Copies of police or U.S. Coast Guard reports
- Paramedic dispatch logs

Table of Contents and Index

Your report should have both a table of contents and an index, so it is easy for the reader to find information quickly. Most word processors and all page layout programs can help you to easily generate these two sections of your report.

Confidentiality of Findings

It should go without saying that information gathered during your investigation is considered confidential. It can only be shared with people who have a legal right to access this information.

If you are conducting an insurance investigation for a recreational diving training agency or a commercial diving firm, in most cases, the attorney who is handling the case will not want you to give a copy of the report to the insured party. If this is done, this makes your findings discoverable in court.

Maintaining Files

All of the original information that you collect, as well as a copy of your report, should be stored in a safe place, for a period of at least seven years following your investigation. It's not uncommon for an investigator to be called on to clarify information in the file long after the investigation is complete.

If you are called to court to testify as to your findings, you'll need access to all of your data to prepare for your testimony. Be sure to file your investigations in a manner that makes it easy to access the information you need.

Testimony

While it is rare for most diving accident investigators to be required to testify in a diving accident case, it does happen. In most civil cases, the attorneys handling the case will only have their experts provide testimony.

When you are required to testify as an investigator, you must be properly prepared. Your preparation should include an exhaustive review of your report, as well as a review of the raw data that you used to create your report. Carefully look over any photographs, video, autopsies, police documents, and anything else that is in your file.

Probably the best preparation that you can perform is to anticipate the type of questions that you feel you will be asked, write them down, and then prepare your response. Rehearse your responses by role playing with a trusted friend or family member.

When you testify in court, you want to make your answers as brief as possible, preferably replying with only a "yes" or a "no." Always pause before answering

National Compressed Air Certification

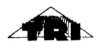

TRI/ENVIRONMENTAL, INC.
A Texas Research International Company
9063 Bee Caves Road • Austin, Texas 78733-6201
(512)263-2101 • (800)880-8378
Fax: (512)263-2558

MARINE MARKETING
ATTN: STEVE BARSKY

FOR:

ANALYSIS RESULTS

ANALYTE	SOURCE AIR	AMBIENT AIR	AIR STANDARD
OXYGEN (%)	20.8	COM#: 05	20-22
CARBON MONOXIDE (ppm)	1.9	COM#: 05	10
METHANE (ppm)	2.1	COM#: 05	N/A
TOTAL GASEOUS HYDROCARBONS (ppm) - METHANE	< 1	COM#: 05	25
CARBON DIOXIDE (ppm)	435	COM#: 05	1000
OIL MIST & PARTICULATE (mg/m^3)	N/A	N/A	5

REPORT NUMBER: 99-11692XREPORT DATE: 12/07/1999   CUSTOMER NO.:A0361
AIR SOURCE: SCUBA CYLINDER   SAMPLE DATE: 12/03/1999
AIR SAMPLED FROM: CYLINDER   KIT NO.:   241
COMPARED TO AIR STANDARD: CGA Type I Grade E
ANALYZED BY: M. MONTGOMERY
USING: 70SOP-36 REV1 & 70SOP-41 REV0 GC: 70-09 BALANCE : 70-03
SB: 25891 AB: 20256 FT: 0 MO: 0

*This is not a complete analysis; only gases analyzed.
<0b> Gas only sample spare bottle. Results not reported.

Fig. 14.6 Make sure you maintain complete copies of all of the documents in your investigation for at least seven years.

any question to allow time for the attorney with whom you are working to raise an objection. It's up to judge to decide whether the question stands or not.

You should not give long winded answers, nor do you want to volunteer any information. You must only answer the precise question that was asked.

It is extremely important during your testimony that you do not appear as an advocate for either side, but that you take a neutral position, no matter what your personal opinions about the case might be. As an investigator, your job is to supply the facts of your investigation, not to render an opinion, which is the role of an expert witness.

Case History – Recreational Diving

A husband and wife were taking a deep diving class from a diving instructor at a freshwater quarry on the east coast. The quarry is known to have poor visibility at depth, but was a convenient training site and a popular local attraction.

The quarry has steeply sloping sides that drop off into waters that are over 300 feet deep. Mud and silt line the bottom and sides of the quarry.

The dive went smoothly for the first 15 minutes until the husband began to run low on air. At that point the instructor gave both divers the signal to ascend. As they started up from the bottom, the wife was making a proper ascent, while the husband appeared to be in difficulty, stirred up the silt, and disappeared in the murk.

The instructor was in a dilemma, whether to continue to make a normal ascent with the wife, or to take off after the missing husband. Rather than risk injury to both divers, the instructor started to ascend with the wife, hoping that once they rose above the silt, he would be able to see the bubbles from the missing diver and go to his aid. As they reached a depth of 50 feet, the instructor spotted a few bubbles rising from the bottom. He sent the wife to the surface by herself, and started back down to the bottom, but had insufficient air to conduct an effective search.

Back on the surface, the instructor immediately called 911 and the local sheriff's dive team was dispatched to look for the missing man. They were unable to locate him after several hours of searching. The body was not discovered for two weeks, at which time it was brought to the surface.

When the dive computer from the missing diver was downloaded to a PC, the resulting dive profile showed a highly compressed version of the time frame of the original dive. This was because the dive computer had been running continuously underwater for two weeks so the data points were pushed closely together. This led to some speculation on the part of the sheriff's department that the dive instructor was not telling the truth, and that perhaps the victim had actually been murdered. The analysis by the dive accident investigator, who was familiar with the behavior of the dive computer under these circumstances, was given to the sheriff's detective. The dive instructor was exonerated from any wrongdoing, based on the investigator's report.

Notes:

Recommendations to Help Avoid Commercial Diving Accidents

1. Follow the Association of Diving Contractors Consensus Standards religiously. Don't just pay lip service to things like the Job Hazard Analysis. Perform a Job Hazard Analysis and follow its dictates.

2. Make sure you are in compliance with all relevant government standards, including OSHA and the U.S. Coast Guard, as well as your own company safety manual.

3. Maintain good records on all of your equipment. Know when each piece of gear was purchased or went into service. Keep accurate records for all maintenance and testing.

4. Perform regularly scheduled maintenance and equipment tests.

5. Don't neglect diving physicals for all diving personnel. Be sure to have a baseline employment physical done, even if a diver comes to you with a "recent" physical from another employer.

6. Have safety officers regularly spot check dive logs to ensure that proper decompression procedures have been followed. Make sure every dive is logged and the diving safety manual is always on site.

7. Use appropriate guards when using power equipment and water blasters.

8. Don't allow a diver to use the wrong tool for a particular job even if it saves time. Always use the right tool for the job.

9. If the diver provides his own helmet, make sure that the maintenance on it is current and that it is in proper working condition prior to any dive. If the company supplies the helmet, any repair or maintenance should be performed by factory authorized technicians.

10. Make sure that only the original manufacturer's parts are used any time a repair is done on a piece of diving or support equipment.

11. If you hire someone with a drug or alcohol problem, without performing a background check or drug screening, that employee's problem becomes your problem.

12. A dive is a dive, whether it's done in 5 feet of water or 500 feet of water. Treat every dive as a serious event.

13. Be sure to have an evacuation plan for injured personnel, which includes names and contact information for facilities and individuals that might be needed in an emergency.

About the Authors

Steven M. Barsky

Steve Barsky started diving in 1965 in Los Angeles County, and became a diving instructor in 1970. His first employment in the industry was with a dive store in Los Angeles and he went on to work for almost 10 years in the retail dive store environment.

Steve attended the University of California at Santa Barbara, where he earned a Masters Degree in 1976 in Human Factors Engineering. This has greatly assisted his thorough understanding of diving equipment design and use. His master's thesis was one of the first to deal with the use of underwater video systems in commercial diving. His work was a pioneering effort at the time (1976) and was used by the Navy in developing applications for underwater video systems.

His background includes being a commercial diver; working in the offshore oil industry in the North Sea, Gulf of Mexico, and South America. He worked as both an air diving supervisor and a mixed-gas saturation diver, making working dives down to 580 feet.

Barsky was marketing manager for Viking America, Inc., an international manufacturer of dry suits. He also served in a similar position at Diving Systems International, now called Kirby Morgan Dive Systems, Inc., the world's leading manufacturer of commercial diving helmets. At DSI, Barsky worked very closely with Bev Morgan, a diving pioneer.

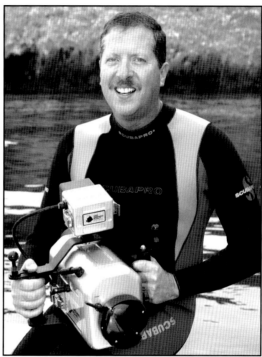

Steve Barsky prepares to dive at Anacapa Island.

Steve is an accomplished underwater photographer. His photos have been used in numerous magazine articles, catalogs, advertising, training programs, and textbooks.

A prolific writer, Barsky's work has been published in *Sea Technology, Underwater USA, Skin diver, Offshore Magazine, Emergency, Fire Engineering, Dive Training Magazine, Searchlines, Sources, Undersea Biomedical Reports, Santa Barbara Magazine, Selling Scuba, Scuba Times, Underwater Magazine*, and many other publications.

About the authors

He is the author of the *Dry Suit Diving Manual, Diving in High-Risk Environments, Spearfishing for Skin and Scuba Divers, Small Boat Diving, Diving with the EXO-26 Full Face Mask, Diving with the Divator MK II Full Face Mask, The Simple Guide to Snorkeling Fun,* and a joint author with Dick Long and Bob Stinton of *Dry Suit Diving: A Guide to Diving Dry.* Steve has taught numerous workshops on contaminated water diving, dry suits, small boat diving, spearfishing, and other diving topics. With his wife Kristine, he wrote *California Lobster Diving* and *Careers in Diving* (with Ronnie Damico).

In 1989 Steve formed Marine Marketing and Consulting, based in Santa Barbara, California. The company provides market research, marketing plans, consulting, newsletters, promotional articles, technical manuals, and other services for the diving and ocean industry. He has consulted to Dräger, AquaLung/U.S. Divers Co., Inc, Zeagle Systems, Inc., Diving Unlimited Intnl., Diving Systems Intnl., DAN, NAUI, and numerous other companies. He also investigates diving accidents and serves as an expert witness in dive accident litigation. He has taught specialized diving courses for organizations like Universal Studios, the U.S. Bureau of Reclamation, the City of San Diego Lifeguards, the National Park Service, and the American Academy of Underwater Sciences.

In 1999 Steve and his wife Kristine formed Hammerhead Press to publish high quality diving books. Both Marine Marketing and Consulting and Hammerhead Press operate under the umbrella of the Carcharodon Corporation.

In 2001, Steve wrote and produced four books for Scuba Diving International; *Deeper Sport Diving with Dive Computers - Wreck, Boat, and Drift Diving - Easy Nitrox Diving -* and *Underwater Navigation, Night, and Limited Visibility Diving.*

Steve is also a partner in Scuba-Training.Net, one of the first on-line distance training programs in the scuba industry. The web site provides the academic portion of diver training including text, photos, animations, and full-motion videos. Both quizzes and exams are administered and graded instantly on the site.

Steve has produced several video projects including a CD-ROM for Viking dry suits and a DVD on California Lobster Diving. Both of these projects were produced by Hammerhead Video.

Steve lives in Ventura, California, with his wife Kristine, and they regularly dive at the Channel Islands.

Tom S. Neuman, M.D., FACP, FACPM
Director, Hyperbaric Medicine Center
Professor of Medicine and Surgery
University of California, San Diego

Dr. Neuman was trained as a Naval Undersea Medical Officer, and has made many original contributions to the field of diving medicine and physiology. He was an undersea medical officer for such diverse commands as Submarine Development Group One, UDT/SEAL PAC 1/3/5, and Harbor Clearance Unit ONE. He retired from the Naval Reserve in 1996.

Dr. Neuman was President of the Undersea and Hyperbaric Medical Society in 1989. Dr. Neuman has been a member of the San Diego County coroner's committee to investigate diving deaths since 1974 and has an extensive experience investigating the medical aspects of diving accidents for multiple governmental and private organizations. His most recent work has been on the diagnosis of decompression sickness and arterial gas embolism.

He has published extensively in the field of the pathophysiology of arterial gas embolism and is interested in the relationship between diving accidents and asthma as well as the mechanism of death associated with arterial gas embolism. He was the Editor-in-Chief of the *Journal of Undersea and Hyperbaric Medicine* from 1995-2002. He is also one of the editors of the *5th Edition of Bennett and Elliott's Physiology and Medicine of Diving* which is

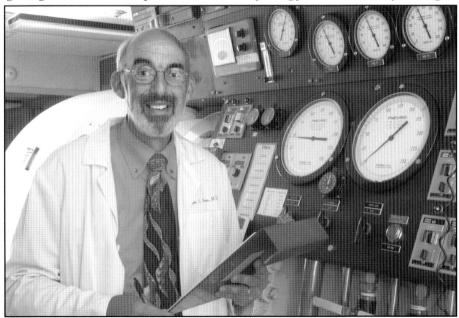

Dr. Tom Neuman at the U.C. San Diego Hyperbaric Medicine Center.

one of three leading textbooks in the field of diving medicine. This was published in January 2003.

Dr. Neuman is on the American Board of Preventive Medicine committee responsible for formulating the Board Examination in Undersea and Hyperbaric Medicine and he is also the American College of Emergency Physician's liaison to that committee. Dr. Neuman is a consultant to NASA and was a member of an Institute of Medicine (IOM) Committee on the medical aspects of exploratory class deep space missions which resulted in the IOM publication *Safe Passage: Astronaut Care for Exploration Missions.* He is a member of an IOM standing committee to advise NASA on extreme environments and medical planning for astronaut health care.

Dr. Neuman is an active diver and an "emeritus" PADI Instructor (#1149). He is board certified in internal medicine, pulmonary medicine, emergency medicine, undersea and hyperbaric medicine, and preventive medicine. He is currently on the full time faculty of the University of California San Diego, where he is the Associate Director of Emergency Medical Services and is the director of the Hyperbaric Medicine Program.

Bibliography

Alexander, A. *Diving Law Update,* in Underwater Magazine, Houston, TX, Spring, 1999, pg. 97-98

American Bureau of Shipping. *Rules for Building and Classing Underwater Vehicles, Systems, and Hyperbaric Facilities, 2003.* ABS, Houston, TX. 2002

Association of Diving Contractors International. *Consensus Standards for Commercial Diving and Underwater Operations, Fifth Edition.* Best Publishing Company, Flagstaff, AZ. 2003

Bachrach, A., and Egstrom, G. *Stress and Performance in Diving.* Best Publishing Company, San Pedro, CA. 1987

Barsky, S. *Diving in High-Risk Environments, Third Edition.* Hammerhead Press, Santa Barbara, CA. 1999

Barsky, S. *Dry Suit Diving, Third Edition.* Hammerhead Press, Santa Barbara, CA. 1999

Caruso, J.L., Bove, A.A. Uguccioni, D.M., Ellis, J.E., Dovenbarger, J.A., and Bennett, P.B. *Recreational diving deaths associated with cardiovascular disease: epidemiology and recommendations for pre-participation screening.* Undersea and Hyperbaric Medicine 28 (suppl) 75. Bethesda, MD 2001

Bozanic, J. *Mastering Rebreathers.* Best Publishing Co., Flagstaff, AZ. 2002

Chowdhury, B. *The Last Dive.* Harper Collins Publishers. New York, NY. 2000

DiMaio, V., and Dana, S. *Forensic Pathology.* Landes Bioscience, Austin, TX. 1998

Divers Alert Network. *Report on Diving Accidents and Fatalities, 1996 Edition.* Divers Alert Network, Durham, NC. 1996

Divers Alert Network. *Report on Diving Accidents and Fatalities, 1997 Edition.* Divers Alert Network, Durham, NC. 1997

Divers Alert Network. *Report on Decompression Illness and Diving Fatalities, 2000 Edition.* Divers Alert Network, Durham, NC. 2000

Dix, J., Graham, M., and Hanzlick, R. *Asphyxia and Drowning: An Atlas.* CRC Press, New York, NY. 2000

Flook, V., and Brubakk, A. *Lung Physiology and Diver's Breathing Apparatus.* University of Aberdeen, Aberdeen, Scotland. 1995

Gerber, S. *The Pathology of Homicide.* Charles C. Thomas, Springfield, IL. 1974

McBride, W. *High Pressure Breathing Air Handbook.* Sub-Aquatics, Inc. 1996

Neuman, T., and Brubakk, A. (Editors),*Bennett and Elliott's Physiology and Medicine of Diving, 5th Edition.* Saunders. London, England. 2003

Nuckols, M., Tucker, W., and Sarich, A. *Life Support Systems Design.* Simon & Schuster Custom Publishing. Needham Heights, MA. 1996

O'Neill, J. *Safety Consideration in Undersea Life Support* in "Proceedings of the Working Diver Symposium," 1974. Batelle Institute, Columbus, OH. 1974

Poynter, D. *The Expert Witness Handbook.* Para Publishing, Santa Barbara, CA. 1987

Richter, E. Friedman, L., Tamir, Y., Berman, T. Levy, O., Westin, J., and Peretz, T. *Cancer Risks in Naval Divers with Multiple Exposures to Carcinogens.* Hebrew University, Jerusalem, Israel. 2002

Tang, K., and Chong, P. *Skilled Labor Worklife and Benefit: A Case Study of Divers in Oil and Gas Exploration.* Dept. of Quantitative Business Analysis, Louisiana State University, Baton Rouge, LA. 1993

Teather, Robert. *The Underwater Investigator.* Best Publishing, Flagstaff, AZ. 1994

Truxillo, D. *Seaman Status, Divers: A Legal Brief* in Underwater Magazine, Summer, 1995, Houston, TX pg. 40

U.S. Coast Guard. *Navigation Rules: International-Inland.* U.S. Department of Transportation, Washington, DC. 1989

Workman, W. *Hyperbaric Facility Safety: A Practical Guide.* Best Publishing Company, Flagstaff, AZ. 1999

Index

Index

Index

R

rack 65

rack operator 65, 188, 189, 191

rapid ascent 180

rebreather 27, 55, 56, 83, 85, 175

receipts 116

recertification 178

records 123, 132

recreation 26, 29

recreational diver 37, 59, 89, 139, 141, 143, 173

recreational diving 18, 25, 28, 37, 40, 44, 55, 62, 112, 119

recreational scuba training 177

red-tag 198

reef 81, 91

regulations 18, 19

regulator 27, 29, 37, 38, 46, 48, 49, 50, 51, 52, 57, 58, 60, 61, 64, 66, 93, 140, 156, 159, 160, 161, 163, 165, 166, 168, 171

regulator performance 51

release 111, 170

release of liability 125

relief valve 45, 61, 63, 69

remote exhaust 46

rental gear 41, 162, 169, 196

rental marking 162, 168

rental record 116, 161

repair department 123

repeating event 105

report 19, 20, 93, 95, 96, 97, 101, 104, 105, 106, 108, 109, 205, 206, 207, 208, 209, 210, 211, 212, 214

reporter 208

reputation 160

rescue 184, 199

rescuer 112

rescue agencies 205

rescue buoy 148

reserve 47, 48, 62

resistance 50, 51

resolution 102

response log 115

retailer 87

retractors 106

Richter, Dr. Elihu 196

rig fire 71

ring 48, 49

rocks 138, 143

roster 124

rough sea 201

ROV 197

rubber parts 51

rubber shroud 161

ruler 169

Rule 27 73, 74

S

safe-second 50

safety 55, 56, 58, 59, 65, 70, 184, 185, 186, 191, 195

safety diver 25, 26, 31

safety line 141

safe deposit box 123

salt water 51

salvage 72

sand 51, 164

sanitation 71, 73

saturation diving 25, 29, 32,33, 43, 71, 73, 189, 190, 191, 194, 202

saturation diving supervisor 187

saturation storage depth 33

saturation system 25, 33, 71

saturation technician 93

scanner 101, 104

scanning software 104

scientific diver 20, 25, 37, 56, 84, 138, 173, 174, 175

scientific diving course 173

scientist 112

scuba 25, 26, 27, 28, 29

scuba cylinder 38, 45, 47, 48, 49, 50, 57, 61, 62, 170

scuba experience 146

scuba retailer 80

seafood diver 17, 20, 183, 184, 185, 201

seal 38, 41, 42, 50, 58, 72, 164

seasonal personnel 183

seawater 139, 149

seaweed 59

sea level 139

sea urchin 29, 35

second stage 29

security 104

seizure 84, 181

self contained underwater breathing apparatus (scuba) 25, 26, 27, 28, 29

semi-closed circuit rebreather 27, 113

sequence of events 96

serial number 106, 107, 161, 164, 165, 166, 168, 169

series of dives 52

sewer outfall 183

sexual harassment 153, 156

shark 143

shift 187, 188, 189, 190, 194

232